SURGERY - PROCEDURES, COMPLICATIONS, AND RESULTS

ARTHROSCOPY: TYPES, PROCEDURES AND RISKS

SURGERY - PROCEDURES, COMPLICATIONS, AND RESULTS

Additional books in this series can be found on Nova's website under the Series tab.

Additional E-books in this series can be found on Nova's website under the E-book tab.

SURGERY - PROCEDURES, COMPLICATIONS, AND RESULTS

ARTHROSCOPY: TYPES, PROCEDURES AND RISKS

KRITON ELANI

AND

HENRI ARVIDSSON

EDITORS

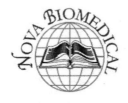

Nova Biomedical Books

New York

For permission to use material from this book please contact us:
Telephone 631-231-7269; Fax 631-231-8175
Web Site: http://www.novapublishers.com

NOTICE TO THE READER

LIBRARY OF CONGRESS CATALOGING-IN-PUBLICATION DATA

Arthroscopy : types, procedures, and risks / editors, Kriton Elani and Henri Arvidsson.
    p. ; cm.
 Includes bibliographical references and index.
 ISBN 978-1-61470-955-8 (softcover)
 1. Arthroscopy. 2. Surgery--Complications. I. Elani, Kriton. II. Arvidsson, Henri.
 [DNLM: 1. Arthroscopy. 2. Intraoperative Complications. 3. Postoperative Complications.
WE 304]
 RD686.A78 2011
 617.4'720597--dc23
                              2011028035

Published by Nova Science Publishers, Inc. † New York

Contents

Preface

Arthroscopy is a minimally invasive surgical procedure in which an examination and sometimes treatment of damage of the interior of a joint is performed using an arthroscope, a type of endoscope that is inserted into the joint through a small incision. In this book, the authors present topical research in the study of the types, procedures and risks of arthroscopy. Topics discussed include arthroscopic rotator cuff repair; indications and techniques for hip arthroscopy; arthroscopic repair of avulsed triangular fibrocartilage complex to the fovea of the distal ulna; arthroscopic lysis and lavage in Wilkes Stage III and IV disease and office-based knee arthroscopy.

Chapter I - Tendon has unique structural properties allowing it to handle high uni-directional loads combined with an ability to stretch and recoil efficiently. This is due to the high proportion of parallel-orientated type 1 collagen bundles, ground substance and elastin. The Insertion of the tendon into the humerus is histologically divided into four zones; tendon, unmineralised fibrocartilage, mineralized fibrocartilage and bone.

Chapter II - From its infancy in the 1950s onwards [1], arthroscopic instrumentation and technique has evolved exponentially. An increasing number of procedures are performed arthroscopically through the increasing sophistication of surgical equipment and the heightened awareness and education amongst the orthopaedic community. This has led to the arthroscopic treatment of a greater range of joints and pathologies. Compared to conventional open surgical procedures, arthroscopic procedures are less likely to result in complications connected to the necessity for larger incisions. They are less invasive for patients and may result in a lower chance of infection, less postoperative pain and faster repair following surgery. There are obvious benefits to the patient and through better health economics, the whole community.

Chapter III - Hip arthroscopy has evolved from an experimental and mainly diagnostic tool, to a standard and effective surgical procedure for the diagnosis and treatment of a variety of disorders not only within but outside the hip as well. The procedure allows for a less invasive approach leading to a faster recovery and decreased peri-operative morbidity compared with the alternative approach of exposing the joint via surgical dislocation of the hip. Furthermore, the recent discovery of Femoroacetabular impingement (FAI) coupled with the surge of interest in sports surgery around the hip has led to improvement of techniques in clinical examination around the hip and imaging as well. This has meant that conditions which were previously unrecognized are being described and can be effectively treated with hip arthroscopy. However, the procedure has a long learning curve, requires appropriate training and specialized equipment and is not for the occasional operator. The results of surgery are dependent on careful patient selection and meticulous pre-operative planning. The aim of this chapter, therefore, is present to the reader a systematic approach to history, clinical examination and investigations of a young adult with hip pain, a detailed account of the technical aspects of hip arthroscopy, the indications for which it is useful along with the possible complications and contraindications. Finally, a brief description of the current research in the authors' departments and future developments of this exciting procedure will be discussed.

Chapter IV - The triangular fibrocartilage complex (TFCC) plays an important role in stabilizing the distal radioulnar joint (DRUJ) during forearm rotation. Therefore, tears of the TFCC lead to varying degrees of DRUJ instability and to symptomatic conditions of the wrist. The ulnar end of the TFCC consists of 3 components, including the proximal triangular ligament, the distal hammock structure, and the ulnar collateral ligament. Among the 3 components, the proximal triangular ligament represents the deep component (dc-TFCC) inserting into the fovea adjacent to the articular surface of the distal ulna (ulnar fovea). Recent anatomical and biomechanical studies have demonstrated that the TFCC insertion into the fovea of the distal ulna has a greater effect on DRUJ stability than other insertion sites. Therefore, surgical reattachment against avulsion of the foveal TFCC insertion must be considered to achieve stability for the DRUJ. Although open techniques of reattachment for avulsed dc-TFCC to the ulna have been introduced, arthroscopic repair techniques have not been established because of technical difficulties. To address this concern, the authors developed a new technique of arthroscopic reattachment of the avulsed dc-TFCC into the ulnar fovea. In this chapter, they mainly introduce previous open and their arthroscopic procedures for the treatment of this lesion.

Chapter V - *Purpose:* To evaluate the analgesic efficacy and function after a single intra-articular (i.a.) injection of sodium hyaluronate (SH) (1 ml at 1%) into temporomandibular joint (TMJ) as a complement to arthroscopic lysis and lavage in Wilkes stage III and IV disease. *Patients and Methods:* A comparative, randomized, double-blind, pilot controlled clinical trial was performed. Forty patients with an internal disorder of the TMJ (Wilkes III-IV) with joint pain and/or mouth-opening limitation were randomly assigned to 2 groups of 20. The experimental group received Ringer lactate plus an injection of 1 ml of SH in the superior joint space of the TMJ after arthroscopy, whereas the control group was given Ringer lactate without viscoelastic supplementation during arthroscopy. Clinical evaluation was carried out using a visual analogue scale (VAS) on the pain and joint function criteria. A secondary evaluation examined disc position and tolerance of treatment. The patients were followed up for 6 months with five assessments. Suitable parametric and nonparametric statistic tests were performed, and the level of statistical significance was set at .05. *Results:* The reduction in joint pain was statistically significant in the treatment group with respect to the control group on the visits on days 14 and 84. Compared to baseline, the level of analgesia was statistically significant in the treated group on day 28. The tolerance of treatment was considered optimal in the control and experimental groups. *Conclusion:* An i.a. injection of SH following arthroscopic lysis and lavage is effective in reducing pain in patients with TMJ dysfunction. Furthermore, SH enhances post-surgical recovery. The analgesic effect of treatment with SH is maintained in the long term.

Chapter VI - Although arthroscopy has a low degree of invasiveness, it still requires considerable time, cost, and effort to be perfomed in the operating room. Surgeons or patients sometimes hesitate due to risks and constrains, especially for a diagnostic second-look arthroscopy. In order to make knee arthroscopy less invasive, the authors use a 1.9 mm–diameter scope. The purpose of this study is to assess the feasibility and usefulness of this method for diagnostic knee arthroscopy without using the operating room. Local anesthesia is placed at the lateral infrapatellar portal, and the joint is inflated. Skin and capsule are penetrated directly by the apex of the obturator, and the scope is inserted into the joint. Saline irrigation is used during arthroscopic evaluation. The wound is closed by a bandage, without need for suture. Video images obtained during arthroscopy were reviewed by three orthopaedic surgeons. The images were scored based on the classification from three categories: 3 points, useful; 2 points, somewhat useful; 1 point, useless. The average point was used for the final evaluation. The patients assessed pain with a visual analog scale (100 mm long from no pain [0] to unbearable pain [100]). Twenty patients were reviewed on this cliteria. Video images were evaluated as 3 points for fifteen patients, as 2.7 points for three and 2.3 points for two patients. Mean pain score was 13.4 mm. Downsizing the scope allows the procedure to be done simply as insertion and removal without incision or suture, reducing risk of infection. This technique makes diagnostic arthroscopy feasible in the office of clinic without using the operating room and increases the likelihood of direct observation of the joint whenever the surgeon or patient feels it necessary. Thus, this method is especially useful for second-look diagnosis of cartilage in settings such as post-cartilage repair.

Chapter VII - ACL (anterior cruciate ligament) partial tears include various types of lesions and an high rate of these lesions evolve into complete tears. Most of the techniques described in literature for the surgical treatment of chronic partial ACL tears, don't spare the intact portion of the ligament. Aim of this study was to perform a prospective analysis of the results obtained by augmentation surgery using gracilis and semitendinosus tendons to treat partial sub-acute lesions of the ACL. This technique requires an "over the top" femoral passage, which enables salvage and strengthening of the intact bundle of ACL. The study included 89 patients treated consecutively at the authors' Institute from 1993 to 2003 with a mean injury-surgery interval of 21 weeks (12 - 39). Patients were followed up by clinical and instrumental assessment criteria at 3 months, 1 year and 5 years after surgery. Clinical assessment was performed with the IKDC form. Subjective and functional parameters were assessed by the Tegner activity scale. Instrumental evaluation was done using the KT-2000 instrument: the 30 pound passive test and the manual maximum displacement test were performed. The authors obtained good to excellent results in 96.6% of cases. They didn't observed recurrences in ligamentous laxity. The authors believe that the described technique has the advantage of being little invasive, compatible with the ACL anatomy, and enables very rapid functional recovery and return to sport.

In: Arthroscopy
Editors: K. Elani et al.

ISBN: 978-1-61470-955-8
© 2012 Nova Science Publishers, Inc.

Chapter I

Arthroscopic Rotator Cuff Repair: Where Are We Now?

S. B. M. MacLean and M. Snow
Royal Orthopaedic Hospital NHS Foundation Trust, Birmingham,
United Kingdom

THE ROTATOR CUFF PROPERTIES AND TIMING OF SURGERY

Tendon has unique structural properties allowing it to handle high uni-directional loads combined with an ability to stretch and recoil efficiently. This is due to the high proportion of parallel-orientated type 1 collagen bundles, ground substance and elastin.

The Insertion of the tendon into the humerus is histologically divided into four zones; tendon, unmineralised fibrocartilage, mineralized fibrocartilage and bone.

The major arterial supply to the rotator cuff is derived from the ascending branch of the anterior humeral circumflex artery, the acromial branch of the thoracoacromial artery, as well as the suprascapular and posterior humeral circumflex arteries. The pathogenesis of rotator cuff tears has been considered to be influenced by the microvascular supply of the rotator cuff tendons. Most cadaver studies have demonstrated a hypovascular area within the critical zone of the supraspinatus tendon. It has been suggested that this area of hypovascularity has a significant role in the attritional degeneration of the aging tendon. However recent studies support the fact that increased vascularity is a normal response to smaller tears but that as tear size increases, the healing response fails and decreased vascularity is observed. [1]

Most textbooks and anatomical studies state that the supraspinatus inserts into the highest impression of the greater tuberosity and the infraspinatus inserts into the middle impression of the greater tuberosity. Recently however, Sugaya et al [2] dissected the rotator cuffs of 113 cadaveric shoulders. He found that the supraspinatus insertion was triangular, narrow in dimension and was localized to the *anteromedial* area of the highest impression of the greater tuberosity, whilst the infraspinatus occupied the *anterolateral area of the highest impression and all of the middle impression*. There may be a greater degree of infraspinatus involvement therefore, in rotator cuff tears than previously thought. It is thus important to delineate the tendons at the time of surgery, to enable anatomical footprint reconstruction.

There is little evidence that spontaneous healing of rotator cuff tendon occurs in humans. Tendinous units are at risk of tear progression, retraction, denervation, muscle atrophy, and fatty degeneration. As well as structural changes, mechanical changes such as increase in stiffness and loss of elasticity. Muscle atrophy may be an early feature after a tear but the formation of scar tissue appears to be progressive [3]. Some of these changes are believed to be irreversible with irreversible changes occurring between 6-12 weeks following a tear [4]. Ultimately permanent alteration in the tendon and glenohumeral joint may result leading to rotator cuff arthropathy.

The time-dependent nature of rotator cuff degeneration has implications in the timing of surgery. Few studies have looked at timing of surgery and outcome. This may be due to late presentation, the large number of asymptomatic cuff tears, and difficulty in identifying whether a tear is acute or chronic. The distinction between an acute tear, acute symptoms of a chronic tear, or acute extension of a chronic tear may be impossible. In a young patient with a defined episode of trauma, the precipitating insult can be established. In an older patient, the time period in which he or she has been experiencing symptoms may be vague or a lucent interval may even have been present before pain and weakness become significant enough to warrant presentation to a doctor.

In 1983, Bassett et al [5] reviewed the results of 37 patients with open rotator cuff at different periods within a 3-month window, with an average follow-up of seven years. Although pain relief was similar between groups, active post-operative abduction was 168 degrees for those repaired within 3 weeks, and 126-129 degrees for those repaired between 3 weeks to 3 months. Post-operative function was independent of the size of the tear.

Hantes et al [6], compared the clinical and MRI findings between early (mean 12 days) versus delayed (mean 131 days) repair. There were 15 and 20 patients in each group respectively. At 3 years, UCLA score was 31 and 26, and Constant score was 82 and 70 respectively. This difference was statistically significant. Range of motion was also significantly better in the early group. Re-tear on MR was also more frequent in the delayed group (7 patients versus 5).

Petersen et al [7], reviewed the outcome of 36 patients having undergone arthroscopic rotator cuff repair – evaluating outcomes using the UCLA and ASES scores. It was found that outcome scores and active elevation improved similarly in all patients repaired before 4 months irrespective of the size of the tear. Preoperative fatty atrophy of the cuff did not influence outcome. Massive tears repaired after 4 months had the worst outcome.

Overall, the literature seems to lean towards a benefit in early repair of rotator cuff within several weeks of a traumatic tear occurring. Irreversible change in the tendon substance and cuff retraction with loss of elasticity over a period of months makes effective arthroscopic repair more challenging and may be one reason for the inferior results reported.

MINI-OPEN VS ARTHROSCOPIC REPAIR

The gold standard treatment for symptomatic tears of the rotator cuff has historically been an open technique as pioneered by Codman [8]. This was found in subsequent studies to be reliable and reproducible. [9-10] This procedure however, has been associated with prolonged rehabilitation and morbidity such as severe early post-operative pain, deltoid detachment with subsequent weakness and arthrofibrosis. [11] In response, the assisted 'mini-open' or 'portal extension' technique was developed. These have the potential advantage of less deltoid morbidity and have developed results similar to that of open repairs. [12]

Johnson described the first completely arthroscopic rotator cuff repair in 1993. [13] The potential advantages of this procedure include less pain, the ability to treat intra-articular lesions, better cosmesis, less soft-tissue dissection and a lower risk of deltoid detachment. Potential disadvantages include an increased cost, difficulty in repairing larger tears, technical difficulty, and a steep learning curve.

Churchill et al, [14] evaluated the cost and time of rotator cuff surgery within the New York hospital database in 2006. 1,334 mini-open procedures were compared to 3,890 all-arthroscopic procedures. It was found the operative time was significantly shorter in the mini-open group (103 minutes) compared to the arthroscopic group (113 minutes). The mean surgical charges in the mini-open group was $7,841 compared to $8,985 in the arthroscopic group.

In a large meta-analysis in 2007 by Nho et al [15], shoulder outcome scores, range of motion and complication rates were compared between the two groups. 2,576 studies were compared, with those involving a high proportion of massive tears, partial tears or revision operations excluded. Only one of the seven arthroscopic studies had <90% good or excellent results, compared with five of the eight mini-open studies. All studies had a mean postoperative UCLA score of >30. None of the retrospective cohort studies were able to identify a difference between the mini-open and arthroscopic groups. The percentage of patients who were either satisfied or very satisfied after rotator cuff repair appeared to be similar, with a range of 90-100% in the arthroscopic group and 86-100% in the mini-open group. Although few studies in the meta-analysis compared range of motion as an outcome measure, in those that did, the mean post-operative forward flexion ranged from 149.0 – 169.6 degrees for the arthroscopic group and from 155.0 – 173.0 degrees for the mini-open group. The mean post-operative external rotation ranged from 50.0 – 85.7 degrees for the arthroscopic group and from 50.0 – 66.0 degrees for the mini-open group. There was a 3% prevalence of complications in the arthroscopic group and a 6.6% prevalence in the mini-open group. The main complications in both groups were; failed repair needing revision, arthrofibrosis, and post-operative impingement. Overall, the meta-analysis showed a similar functional outcome between groups with a trend towards higher complication rate in the mini-open group.

A later meta-analysis by Morse et al [16], in 2008, used a stricter inclusion criteria, using only level I-III evidence with a minimum one year follow-up. This meta-analysis concluded that there was no significant difference in either functional outcome or complication rates between the arthroscopic and mini-open groups.

More recently, other studies have compared the two groups. Colegate-Stone et al [17] carried out a comparative cohort study of 31 mini-open repairs and 92 arthroscopic repairs. Subjective and objective functional assessment were performed pre- and post-operatively at regular time intervals up to 24 months, using DASH, OSS and the Constant-Murley score. At every time point the arthroscopic group scored better than the mini-open group using each assessment tool. There was a significant difference in pre-operative scores however, with patients in the mini-open group tending to have lower functional scores before surgery compared to those selected for arthroscopic repairs. Recovery from baseline therefore, was found to be similar in either treatment option at 12 months.

Kose et al [18], compared 25 arthroscopic repairs to 25 mini-open repairs at a mean follow-up of 22 and 31 months respectively. There was no significant difference in pre- and post-operative Constant-Murley, UCLA scores and satisfaction levels between the groups. Patients in the mini-open group stayed on average one day longer in hospital than those in the arthroscopic group. The differences between pain scores and post-operative range of movement were not significant.

Kang et al [19], retrospectively analysed 128 patients with chronic small- and medium-sized rotator cuff tears who underwent mini-open (n=63) or arthroscopic repair (n=65). Outcome was assessed using the DASH score, Simple Shoulder Test, VAS pain score, and the SF-36 health survey. At 3 and 6 months, both groups showed similar and statistically significant improvement in all patient-derived outcome parameters except for three SF-36 variables. There was significantly better SF-36 bodily pain scores at 3 months and the VAS pain score at 6 months postoperatively in the arthroscopic group.

Liem et al [20], compared 19 patients with arthroscopic repair with 19 who had a mini-open repair. There was no difference in clinical and structural outcome as seen on MR scanning. The overall Constant score improved from 53.8 to 83.9 in the arthroscopic group and from 53.5 to 83.7 in the mini-open group. Early range of motion did not differ significantly at 6 weeks or 3 months postoperatively. The number of re-tears was 6 (31.6%) in the arthroscopic group and 7 (36.8%) in the mini-open group. This difference was not statistically significant.

Verma et al [21], also used outcome scores and post-operative imaging to assess repair integrity between 38 patients in an arthroscopic repair group and 33 patients in a mini-open group. No statistical difference in ASES scores were found between the groups post-operatively. 24% in the arthroscopic group and 27% in the mini-open group had recurrent or persistent defects on ultrasound at 2 years. This was not statistically significant. Patients with an original tear >3cm were more likely to have a tear at follow-up. Interestingly patients with persistent defects had similar pain and outcome scores to patients with intact repairs.

Pearsall et al [22], has reported results with mid-term follow-up. They compared 27 patients in an arthroscopic group with 25 in a mini-incision group. The average follow-up was 51 months, and there was no significant difference in post-operative outcome scores or range of motion between the groups.

Senior Author's Opinion

It is difficult to obtain a definitive answer from the literature as to which method of treatment is superior. Individual studies on mini-open versus arthroscopic repair are often limited by small numbers in each treatment arm. The larger meta-analyses are limited by the number of different outcome measures used, the variation in inclusion/exclusion criteria and surgical technique making comparison and conclusion difficult. Currently all one can say is that there is no significant difference between the 2 techniques. Whilst the arthroscopic group carries with it slightly increased costs, there is a possible trend towards increased complications in the mini-open group.

It is our personal choice to undertake an all arthroscopic repair. We believe it allows improved visualisation, better evaluation of tear configuration and consequently a more anatomical repair. The arthroscopic enthusiasts (of which I am one) often argue that repairing large/massive tears arthroscopically is where arthroscopy is particulary advantageous, due to better visualisation and the sparing of deltoid. Conversely, the mini-open enthusiasts state that open repairs of small / medium size tears are much quicker and more efficient. If one does not repair the small tears arthroscopically it is difficult to imagine a surgeon developing their skills sufficiently to consistently repair the technically more challenging larger tears.

SINGLE VERSUS DOUBLE-ROW REPAIR

Structural failure and recurrent tears are frequent postoperative problems in rotator cuff repair. The development of a fibrovascular interface between tendon and bone is a requirement for healing, with the possibility of restoring a fibrocartilaginous insertion. Traditional repair techniques utilise a single row repair. In recent years, there has increasing interest in double row repairs. A double row repair uses a row of anchors medially-near the supero-lateral margin of the humeral articular cartilage and a lateral row-near the edge of the cuff insertion on the greater tuberosity. There are a number of different double row configurations, but they can be classified into 2 main types;

- *Double row (DR)* - consists of a row of medial anchors who's sutures have been passed in a mattress fasion and a separate lateral row consisting of simple sutures.
- *Double row suture bridge (DRSB)* - consists of a medial row of anchors and mattress sutures. The tails of the medial row sutures are then passed through either a bone tunnel or a knotless anchor laterally and tensioned to create a compression force over the tendon foot print

It is postulated that a double row repair will allow improved tendon insertion anatomy, with almost 100% coverage of the footprint.

Cadaveric and animal studies have reported the theoretical benefits of double row repair. Kim et al [23] , used 9 matched pairs of cadaveric shoulders, creating a tear in the supraspinatus tendon of each. One group were repaired using a DR repair, and the contralateral with a single row (SR) repair. Each side underwent cyclic loading testing and tensile testing to failure. Gap formation was found to be significantly smaller in the DR repair during loading, and the initial strain in the DR repair was nearly one-third of the SR repair. Adding a medial row of anchors increased the stiffness of the repair by 46% and the ultimate failure load by 48%.

Smith et al [24], used similar methodology in 16 cadaveric shoulders. He found gap formation in the SR group during static loading was significantly greater than the double-row group. Under cyclic loading, the double-row repairs failed at a mean of 320N whereas the SR repairs failed at a mean of 224N.

Grimberg et al [25], studied pressure and contact surface area between SR and DR repairs of supraspinatus in cadaveric specimens. They found that there was a significant increase in contact pressure with double-row repair compared to single-row repair.

Milano et al [26], assessed mechanical behaviour under cyclic loading of single and double-row configurations in porcine shoulders with 2cm infraspinatus tears. Repairs were done either under tension or tension-free.

Single-row tension repairs showed significantly poorer results for all variables considered. Both tension and tension-free double-row repairs performed best for ultimate failure strength and tendon elongation.

Nelson et al [27], compared the biomechanical strength and surface area of repair in six pairs of sheep shoulder using single-row and double-row repairs of infraspinatus tendon. Double-row repair restored a mean surface area of 258mm versus 148mm for the single-row repair. In this study, however, there was no significant difference in strain at the repair site or load to failure.

Brady et al [28], assessed footprint coverage in double row repairs in 26 patients after tying first the lateral row, followed by the medial row. On average, tying only the lateral row (equivalent to a single row repair) left an uncovered area of 52.7%+/- 9.2%. After the medial row was repaired there was *no* residual deficit on the cuff footprint. It would appear from these studies that surface area of repair and repair strength are independent factors in the outcome of repair.

Baums et al [29], considered the mechanical properties of rotator cuff repair in 32 sheep shoulders with different stitch technique and suture and row configuration. The ultimate tensile strength in double-row specimens was significantly higher than in others and there was no difference in using different suture material. Double-row anchor repair using Mason-Allen/medial mattress stitches provides initial strength superior to single-row repair with Mason-Allen stitches under isometric cyclic loading as well as ultimate failure strength.

In these animal and cadaveric studies, overall the benefits of double-row repair over single-row repair in terms of footprint contact and ultimate failure strength has been shown. Trials on patients have been fraught with small numbers in each treatment arm and results have been less conclusive.

Charrouset et al [30], compared 31 patients undergoing double-row repair with 35 undergoing single-row repair. 6 months post-operatively there was no significant difference in Constant Scores between groups. CT-arthrography was used to judge tendon healing and footprint coverage at 6 months. This was judged to be significantly better in the double-row group; being anatomical in 19 patients in the double-row group and 14 in the single-row group.

Franceschi et al [31], made similar conclusions at 2 year follow-up. Comparing 30 patients with single-row repairs and 30 with double-row repairs, he found no difference in UCLA score and range of motion at 2 years between groups. Post-op MR arthrography at 2 years showed a significant difference in tendon healing however, with more patients in the double-row group having an intact cuff at follow-up.

Park et al [32], compared 40 single-row repairs and 38 double-row repairs at 2 years poat-operatively. He found there to be no significant difference in the Constant scores or ASES scores between groups. In sub-group analysis between different sized tears however, he found that patients with large tears (>3cm) in the double-row repair group had significantly better ASES and Constant scores at 2 years.

Grasso et al [33], carried out a randomized control trial (RCT) with 40 patients in the single-row repair group and 40 in the double-row repair group. Univariate and multivariate analysis was carried out a 2 years post-operatively. There was no significant difference between DASH scores, Constant scores and muscle strength between the groups. Only age, gender and baseline strength independently influenced the outcome.

Burks et al [34], conducted an RCT comparing 20 single-row repairs to 20 double-row repairs. At 1 year post-operatively there were no difference in any of the post-operative measures of motion or strength including; UCLA, Constant, ASES and WORC scores. Post-operative MR scans at 6 weeks, 3 months and 12 months showed no significant differences in terms of footprint coverage, tendon thickness and tendon signal between groups.

Pennington et al [35], prospectively compared 54 double-row repairs with 78 single-row Mason-Allen configuration repairs[1]. At 3, 6, 12 and 24 months, UCLA and ASES scores were compared. There was no significant difference between outcome scores between groups. Post-operative MR scan showed a significantly improved healing rate overall in the single-row repair group. In a subset of patients with tears between 2.5 and 3.5 cm there was shown to be an improved rate of healing in the double-row repair group.

The most recent meta-analysis of the literature compared only 6 papers, highlighting the lack of good quality trials comparing the two methods of

---

[1] Senior Author's Opinion: Double row repair is our preferred technique due to its bio-mechanical benefits. With the advent of new techniques comes new methods of failure. It would appear that with DR repairs, it is now tendon and biological failure which is the likely reason why we have not seen any clinical improvement. This tells us that if we are going to improve our results we must improve the biology. The avascular degenerate nature of the tendon is now the weakest link in the construct. We believe that when we are able to optimise the healing process then we will see the benefits of DR repair that have been reported in the lab. Corresponding Author: Mr. Vikas Khanduja MBBS, MRCS (G), MSc, FRCS, FRCS (Orth), Consultant Orthopaedic Surgeon, Addenbrooke's – Cambridge University Hospitals, Box 37, Hills Road, Cambridge CB2 0QQ, United Kingdom. Tel: 44 1223 309524. Email: vk29@cam.ac.uk.

repairs. [36] The authors' overall conclusions suggested that there was no significant difference between groups in terms of post-operative clinical outcome scores. There may be a trend towards better outcome with double-row repair for patients with large tears (>3cm), however more studies are needed to substantiate this finding.

THE TREATMENT OF PARTIAL-THICKNESS ROTATOR CUFF TEARS

Although a common cause of shoulder pain and occupational disability, studies have shown a high incidence of asymptomatic partial-thickness tears in individuals on imaging. [37] Partial-thickness tears are regarded as being 2-3 times more prevalent in patients as compared to full-thickness tears. [38]

Debate arises as to the aetiology of partial-thickness tears. There are intrinsic and extrinsic mechanisms postulated. Intrinsic factors include the biomechanical fact that the articular surface of supraspinatus, where most tears are found has an ultimate tensile strength approximately half that of the bursal side. [39] Age-related deterioration in tenocyte numbers, vascularity and healing potential are other intrinsic factors leading to tendinopathy in the cuff. The articular side of the rotator cuff is also poorly vascularised, with a critical zone in the lateral portion of the supraspinatus tendon.

Extrinsic factors include the acromion shape, inferior osteophytes on the acromion or acromioclavicular joint and morphology of the coracoacromial arch, causing impingement of the superior rotator cuff tendons. These factors have yet to be substantiated in clinical trials. Other extrinsic factors causing partial-thickness tears include traumatic injury and glenohumeral instability leading to impaired rotator force coupling and subsequent tendinopathy.

Partial thickness tears are more prevalent in younger patients compared with full-thickness tears. Their natural history is unclear. Although they may retain some potential for repair, a prospective arthrographic study found that 1 year after initial evaluation, half of the examined partial thickness tears had become larger, and 25% had progressed to a full thickness tear. [40]

Fiercely debated is the proposed treatment methods for partial-thickness tears. Patients with minimal symptoms usually self-select non-surgical treatment. Initial treatment modalities may include a steroid injection to alleviate inflammatory symptoms, ice, heat and ultrasonography, to decrease pain and muscle spasm. Targeted strength training of the cuff muscles and external muscles of the shoulder girdle may follow. Eccentric and plyometric exercises for the athlete or high-demand individual may be necessary.

Surgical treatment may consist of tendon debridement or tendon repair. Recent literature debates the indications and the results of these treatment methods.

Many papers have correlated the size of the tear to surgical outcome. Mazzocca et al [41], conducted a cadaveric study, creating a partial thickness tear of the supraspinatus tendon of various depths on 20 shoulders. He then carried out strain testing to the torn tendon at different angles of loading and repeated this after an anchor repair. There was found to be a significant difference in rotator cuff strain between the intact tendon and 50% and 75% partial-thickness tears. Cuff stain was returned to normal following repair. Yang et al [42] created bursal-sided partial thickness tears in fresh-frozen shoulder specimens. He dynamically loaded the torn tendon, recording strain. Strain in the intact tendon increased in the intact tendon in a linear fashion, until tear depth reached 50% or greater. At this depth, plastic deformation occurred, and the tear propagated. These studies highlighted the importance of considering surgical repair in tears of 50% or greater of the tendon substance.

Park et al [43] evaluated outcome after arthroscopic debridement in partial thickness tears with a tear depth of less than 50%. 24 articular and 13 bursal partial thickness tears were evaluated for pain relief and functional recovery. At 6 months postoperatively, the average pain score decreased from 6.2 to 1.7 in patients with articular surface tears and from 7.1 to 0.9 in patients with bursal partial thickness rotator cuff tears.

Liem et al [44], prospectively reviewed outcome in 46 partial thickness tears of 50% or less, treated with subacromial decompression. At an average follow-up of 50.3 months the average ASES scores significantly improved from 37.4 to 86.6 points, The mean postoperative Constant score was 87.6 points. Only three patients (6.5%) progressed to a full-thickness tear detectable on ultrasound scan. Overall clinical outcome was rated excellent in 35 cases (76.1%), good in 5 (10.9%), average in 2(4.3%) and poor in 4(8.7%).

Some studies have treated partial thickness tears with debridement only independent of the size of the tear. Snyder et al [45] treated 31 symptomatic partial thickness tears with arthroscopic debridement of the lesion or subacromial decompression. Neer's criteria and the UCLA rating scale were used. 84% of the patients had satisfactory results with the remaining 16% having unsatisfactory results. Lesion size was found to be independent of outcome, and in 3 patients who had repeat arthroscopy there was found to be no progression of the tear.

Reynolds et al [46], assessed the outcome of arthroscopic debridement of small partial thickness tears in professional baseball pitchers. 51 out of the 67 patients (76%) were able to return to competitive pitching and 37 (55%) were able to return to the same level or higher.

Repair of partial tears appear to perform well when compared to full thickness tears. Park et al [47], reviewed the results of arthroscopic repair for

partial- and full-thickness tears. 42 patients were followed-up for 2 years (22 partial-thickness and 20 full thickness tears). At final follow-up average pain scores and functional outcome score were not significantly different.

Deutsch [48] prospectively evaluated the clinical outcome of 41 patients who underwent arthroscopic repair of a significant (>50%) partial thickness tear of supraspinatus. At a mean follow-up of 38 months, postoperative isometric strength measurements revealed no significant difference between the operative and normal shoulders. ASES scores improved from 42 to 93 points, pain relief from 6/5 to 0.8 points, and satisfaction from 3.0 to 9.2 points. Of the 41 patients, 40 (98%) were satisfied with their outcome.

Several studies have compared clinical outcome based on different repair techniques. Spencer et al [49] carried out an 'all-inside repair' for 20 patients with partial thickness tears greater than 50%. This involved a technique that repaired the articular surface tear and did not violate the intact bursal tissue. Postoperative Penn scores improved significantly from 74 to 92 at a mean of 29 months.

Seo et al [50] prospectively reviewed the results of 24 patients with partial thickness tears, all of which had a 'trans-tendon' repair, to attempt to anatomically restore the supraspinatus footprint and avoid 'completing' the tear before repair. At 12 months post-operatively the ASES score significantly improved from 38 to 89, and the VAS scores significantly improved from 6.6 to 0.6. There were no significant differences between the operative and unaffected shoulders at 12 months postoperatively. 22 of 24 patients were either satisfied or very satisfied with postoperative result at 12 months.

A recent systematic review of the literature reviewed 16 studies in which partial thickness tears had been treated with a range of arthroscopic treatment methods [51]. In all 12 studies with available preoperative baseline data, treatment resulted in improved shoulder symptoms and function. For tears greater than 50%, data supported arthroscopic repair, using either arthroscopic takedown and repair, transtendon repairs or transosseus repairs, with all techniques reporting excellent results. In tears less than 50% of the tendon's thickness, debridement +/- subacromial decompression produces good results, although there is a reported 6.5 to 34.6% risk of progression to a full-thickness tear.

AUGMENTATION OF THE ROTATOR CUFF

Between 20-70% of large rotator cuff tears may fail to heal after surgery. This has led to researchers investigating methods to augment the surgical repair of chro that allow it to share the load of the repaired tendon and enable the tendon-graft construct to resist gap formation and failure. Stiffness and a modulus of elasticity similar to that of the intact native tendon are required. The material of the augment should have properties that facilitate healing of the tendon to bone. It must not create a chronic inflammatory response, an allergic or a rejection response from the host. It should have the ability to hold a suture under physiological stress.

Biological patch materials are prepared from extracellular matrix (ECM) of different anatomical origin, and from human or xenogenic origin. Potential advantages of using ECM materials are that they provide an environment conducive to infiltration by recipient cells, revascularization and remodeling into native tissue, as well as providing mechanical support. Xenogenic materials contain the highly antigenic Gal epitope, and although often chemically cross-linked to reduce antigenicity and increase strength, this can result in poor integration and localized inflammation. The results of synthetic and biological patches have been reported in the literature.

Hirooka et al [52], reviewed the effectiveness of augmentation of large cuff repairs using Gore-Tex patches in 27 patients at a mean follow-up of 44 months. The average Japanese Orthopaedic Association Score (JOA) improved from 57.7 to 88.7 points. Average abduction strenth was 6.2kg in the patients who had had a small patch used in comparison to 1.5kg in the large patch group (used in tears >2cm).

Encalada-Diaz et al [53] reviewed ten patients following repair of supraspinatus tendon and augmentation with a polycarbonate polyurethane patch, secured in a 6-point fixation construct placed over the repaired tendon. Patients showed significant improvements in visual analogue pain score, simple shoulder testing, and ASES testing at 6 and 12 months postoperatively. UCLA postoperative scores were good to excellent in 8 patients at 12 months. Range of motion was significantly improved at 6 and 12 months postoperatively. MR imaging showed healing in 90%. No adverse reaction was associated with the patch.

Nada et al [54], reviewed the results of 21 massive chronic rotator cuff tears augmented with a polyester ligament (Dacron) at a mean follow-up of 36 months. All the patients remained free from pain with a significant improvement in function and range of movement. The mean pre-operative and post-operative Constant scores were 46.7 and 85.4 respectively. The mean patient satisfaction score was 90%. There was one failure due to deep infection and one due to a ruptured ligament at one year. The MR scan at final follow-up confirmed intact and thickened bands in 15 of 17 patients.

Several recent studies have looked at the results of using GraftJacket (human dermal ECM) for rotator cuff augmentation. Wong et al [55] reviewed 45 patients with massive rotator cuff tears at a minimum of 2 years following repair and augmentation using GraftJacket. The mean UCLA score increased significantly from 18.4 to 27.5. The average WORC score was 75.2 and the ASES score was 84.1 at the final follow-up.

Bond et al [56], similarly assessed the results of 16 patients with massive contracted tears of the rotator cuff, repaired and augmented with Graftjacket. At a mean follow-up of 26.8 months, 15 of 16 patients were satisfied with the procedure. The mean UCLA score increased from 18.4 to 30.4. The Constant score increased from 53.8 to 84.0. Significant improvements were seen in pain, forward flexion and external rotation strength. 13 patients had full incorporation of the graft into the native tissue as seen on MR scanning. There were no complications reported.

Burkhead et al [57], reported on the use of Graftjacket in the augmentation of rotator cuff repair. 17 patients were followed up for a mean of 14 months, and the functional status of the shoulder evaluated. A significant improvement in UCLA score was found with reduced pain (11 of 17) and improved function (12 of 17) in the majority of the patients. MRI showed graft integration in all cases.

Local autografts can be used to augment repair. Sano et al [58] reported using the intra-articular part of the long head of biceps tendon to augment cuff repair after tenodesis in 14 patients. At a mean follow-up of 28 months average active elevation angle improved from 69-149 degrees. Total JOA score improved from 54.7 to 83.1 points. 13 shoulders showed no re-tearing on MR scan. Bektaser et al [59], reported similar promising results using coracoacomial ligament autograft.

Overall, human-derived matrices are less immunogenic compared to those from animal sources. They have been shown to be mechanically stronger than their synthetic counterparts and serve as a template for the regeneration of human tissue. Although no high quality evidence exists to support the routine use of these grafts thus far, retrospective series and the growing literature suggests that they may perform well in the right circumstances-becoming incorporated into host tissue and improve pain and function post-operatively.

WHAT TO DO WITH THE SUPRASCAPULAR NERVE?

The incidence of suprascapular nerve compression in association with massive rotator cuff tears has been reported to be between 38 and 100%. [60] Post operative analysis of muscle function after complete or partial repair have shown subsequent significant functional improvement in both nerve function and pain. The role of nerve release following repair is unclear, repair itself maybe enough to decompress the nerve. [61] Further studies are needed to determine if nerve release should be carried out routinely in massive tears and in shoulders where repair is not technically possible.

A LOOK TO THE FUTURE – TISSUE ENGINEERING

Age-related tendon degeneration is thought to be due partly to the lack of available tenocytes (differentiated mesenchymal cells in tendon tissue) for repair. Promising studies in animals have looked at the potential of Platelet Rich Plasma (PRP), stem cells, gene-modification and other tissue engineering techniques in repairing the damaged rotator cuff.

Platelet-Rich Plasma

Cytokines from platelets, such as platelet-derived growth factor (PDGF) are known to play an important role in cell chemotaxis, proliferation, matrix synthesis and cell differentiation and may therefore improve rotator tendon-to-bone healing. PRP is a fraction of plasma that has been isolated and used to enhance regeneration in bone and soft tissues. Sub-fractions of PRP, for example the 'Cascade' membrane have been used. This is a thin layer of autologous fibrin, rich in platelets, obtained by high speed centrifugation of a small quantity of PRP. The healing potential of PRP has been attributed to the release of multiple growth factors from the highly concentrated platelets.

Randelli has conducted a randomised controlled trial for the use of PRP [63]. 53 patients who underwent shoulder arthroscopy for the repair of a complete rotator cuff tear were randomly divided into 2 groups (PRP vs control). The pain score in the treatment group was lower than the control group at 3, 7, 14, and 30 days after surgery (P < .05). On the Simple Shoulder Test, UCLA, and Constant scores, strength in external rotation (SER), as measured by a dynamometer, were significantly higher in the treatment group than the control group at 3 months after surgery. There was no difference between the 2 groups after 6, 12, and 24 months. The follow-up MRI showed no significant difference in the healing rate of the rotator cuff tear. In the subgroup of grade 1 and 2 tears, with less retraction, SER in the PRP group was significantly higher at 3, 6, 12, and 24 months postoperative (P < .05).

Castricini et al [64], carried out a randomised controlled trial with 88 patients assigned to receive arthroscopic rotator cuff repair without (n = 45) or with (n = 43) augmentation with autologous platelet-rich fibrin matrix (PRFM). All the patients completed follow-up at 16 months. There was no statistically significant difference in total Constant score when comparing the results of arthroscopic repair of the 2 groups (95% confidence interval, -3.43 to 3.9) (P = .44). There was no statistically significant difference in magnetic resonance imaging tendon score when comparing arthroscopic repair with or without PRFM (P = .07).

Despite the theoretical advantages of PRP, there is an insufficient body of literature to commend its routine use therefore.

Stem Cells and Gene Therapy

Mesenchymal stem cells (MSCs) are multipotent, capable of differentiating into several connective tissue types including osteocytes, chondrocytes, adipocytes, tenocytes and myoblasts. [65] Mesenchymal stem cells have the advantage of being easily obtainable in adult tissue, and with the appropriate microenvironment can differentiate into various target tissue types.

Mazzocca et al, [66] aspirated bone marrow from the bone anchor tunnel in the humeral head during arthroscopic rotator cuff repair in 23 patients. Using a novel device, in the operating room, stem cells were isolated from this aspirate and their presence and osteogenic potential confirmed. This study showed that stem cell-rich bone marrow is exposed following arthroscopic drilling of the humeral head. These stem cells harbour potential to differentiate into ostoblasts and tenocytes to regenerate the bone-tendon interface. Novel solutions for the recruitment and activation of these cells in combination with growth factors, gene therapy and an appropriate scaffold may provide improved strength of the rotator cuff following surgical repair.

Chang et al [67] examined healing potential of infraspinatus tendon in rabbits at the tendinous insertion using a periosteal graft containing autologous MSCs. Histological examination from 4 to 12 weeks showed gradual progression in healing from fibrotic tissue to mineralised fibrocartilage. There was an associated significant increase in failure load with time compared to controls.

Recently Gulotta et al [68] has highlighted the importance of gene expression in stem cells for tendon healing. In a rat supraspinatus model, MSCs after injection were present and metabolically active, but no difference in the biomechanical strength of the repairs, the cross-sectional area, peak stress to failure or stiffness compared to controls could be found. A further study compared an MSC group and a group who had received adenoviral MT1 matrix metalloproteinase-transduced MSCs (Ad-MT1-MMP). Although no difference was found at 2 weeks, at 4 weeks the Ad-MT1-MMP group had significantly more fibrocartilage, higher load to failure, stress to failure and stiffness values as compared to MSCs. [69] It has also been shown that MSCs expressing BMP-2 and the transcription factor Smad8ca leads to differentiation into a tenocyte lineage. [70] It has been proposed that expression of Smad8ca leads to the production of MMPs. Shahab-Osterloh et al [71] showed that MSCs with adenoviral-induced Smad8ca and BMP-2 exhibit both tendinous and osteogenic properties in mice, and can aid formation therefore of bone-tendon interface. Numerous other studies highlight the beneficial effect of BMP in tendon-bone interface healing. [72]

The use of stem cell-coated sutures could have obvious theoretical benefits in surgical repair of the rotator cuff. Yao et al [73] evaluated the fats of pluripotential embryonic stem cells seeded to a suture carrier in acellularised, sectioned rabbit Achilles tendon. At day 5, fluorescence under microscopy showed live metabolically active pluripotential cells at the tendon repair site. The same author showed that cell adherence at seven days was greater in FibreWire sutures when first coated with poly-1-lysine or fibronectin. [74]

Tissue engineering is an exciting developing field that holds promise in the field of regenerative medicine and rotator cuff repair. Studies on human subjects thus far have been limited, but theoretical benefits of the technology are obvious.

SUMMARY

As a major cause of musculoskeletal morbidity, with a huge financial burden to society, there remains much debate as to what constitutes the optimal rotator cuff repair. We have significantly improved our understanding of rotator cuff anatomy and tear patterns over the last 10 years. As a consequence we perform more individualised surgery, resulting in more anatomical tension free repairs. DR repair constructs provide stronger initial repair constructs with great footprint coverage but as yet failed to show a clear clinical benefit. Improvements in biology with the use of therapies such as PRP, stem cells and gene-therapy may hold the key in regenerating tendon and improving functional outcomes.

REFERENCES

[1]   Hegedus EJ, Cook C, Brennan M. Vascularity and Tendon Pathology in the Rotator Cuff: A Review of Literature and Implications for Rehabilitation and Surgery. *Br. J. Sports Med.* 2010; 44(12): 838-847.

[2]   Mochizuki T, Sugaya H, Uomizu M, et al. Humeral insertion of the supraspinatus and Infraspinatus. New anatomical findings regarding the footprint of the rotator cuff. *J. Bone Joint Surg. Am.* 2008; 90: 962-969.

[3]   Buchmann S, Walz L, Sandmann GH, et al. Rotator cuff changes in a full thickness tear rat model: verification of the optimal time interval until reconstruction for comparison to the chronic process of chronic lesions in humans. *Arch. Orthop. Trauma. Surg.* 2011; 131(3): 429-435.

[4]   Gerber C, Meyer DC, Schneeberger AG, et al. Effect of tendon release and delayed repair on the structure of the muscles of the rotator cuff: An experimental study in sheep. *J. Bone Joint Surg. Am.* 2004; 86: 1973-1982.

[5]   Bassett RW, Cofield RH. Acute tears of the rotator cuff. The timing of surgical repair. *Clin. Orthop. Relat. Res*. 1983; 5(175): 18-24.

[6]   Hantes ME, Karidakis GK, Vlychou M, et al. A comparison of early versus delayed repair of traumatic rotator cuff tears. Knee Surg. *Sports Traumatol. Arthrosc. 2011* [Epub – ahead of print].

[7]   Petersen SA, Murphy TP. The timing of rotator cuff repair for the restoration of function. *J. Shoulder Elbow Surg*. 2011; 20(1): 62-68.

[8]   Codman EA. Complete rupture of the supraspinatus tendon: operative treatment with report of two successful cases Boston *Med. Surg. J*. 1911; 164: 708-710.

[9]   Bigliani LU, Cordasco FA, McIlveen et al. Operative repairs of massive rotator cuff tears: long-term results. *J. Shoulder Elbow Surg*. 1992; 1: 120-130.

[10]   Ellman H, Hanker G, Bayer M. Repair of the rotator cuff. End-result study of factors influencing reconstruction. *J. Bone Joint Surg. Am*. 1986; 68(8): 1136-1144.

[11]   Adamson GF, Tibone JE. Ten year assessment of primary rotator cuff repairs. *J. Shoulder Elbow Surg*. 1993; 2: 57-63.

[12]   Levy HJ, Uribe JW Delaney LG. Arthroscopic assisted rotator cuff repair: preliminary results. *Arthroscopy* 1990; 6(1): 55-60.

[13]   Johnson LL. Rotator Cuff. In *Diagnostic and Surgical Arthroscopy of the Shoulder*. Edited by: Johnson LL. St. Louis, Mosby; 1993: 365-405.

[14]   Churchill RS, Ghorai JK. Total cost and operating room time comparison of rotator cuff repair techniques at low, intermediate, and high volume centers: mini-open versus all-arthroscopic. *J. Shoulder Elbow Surg*. 2010; 19(5): 716-721.

[15]   Nho SJ, Shindle MK, Sherman SL, et al. Systematic review of arthroscopic rotator cuff repair and mini-open rotator cuff repair 2001. *J. Bone Joint Surg. Am.;* 89: 127-136.

[16]   Morse K, Davis AD, Afra R et al. Arthroscopic versus mini-open rotator cuff repair: a comprehensive review and meta-analysis. *Am. J. Sports Med*. 2008; 36(9): 1824-1828.

[17]   Colegate-Stone T, Allom R, Tavakkolizadeh A et al. An analysis of outcome of arthroscopic versus mini-open rotator cuff repair using subjective and objective scoring tools. *Knee Surg. Sports Traumatol. Arthrosc*. 2009; 17(6): 691-694.

[18] Kose KC, Tezen E, Cebesoy O, et al/ Mini-open versus all-arthroscopic rotator cuff repair: comparison of the operative costs and the clinical outcomes. *Adv. Ther.* 2008; 25(3): 249-259.

[19] Kang L, Henn RF, Tashjian RZ et al. Early outcome of arthroscopic rotator cuff repair: a matched comparison with mini-open rotator cuff. *Arthroscopy* 20007; 23(6): 573-582.

[20] Liem D, Bartl C, Lichtenberg S, et al. Clinical outcome and tendon integrity of arthroscopic versus mini-open supraspinatus tendon repair: a magnetic resonance imaging-controlled matched-pair analysis. *Arthroscopy* 2007; 23(5): 514-521.

[21] Verma NN, Dunn W, Adler RS et al. All-arthroscopic versus mini-open rotator cuff repair: a retrospective review with minimum 2-year follow-up. *Arthroscopy* 2006; 22(6): 587-594.

[22] Pearsall AW, Ibrahim KA, Madanagopal SG. The results of arthroscopic versus mini-open repair for rotator cuff tears at mid-term follow-up. *J. Orthop. Surg. Res.* 2007; 2(24): 24-32.

[23] Kim DH, Elattrache NS, Tibone JE, et al. Biomechanical comparison of a single-row versus double-row suture anchor technique for rotator cuff repair. *Am. J. Sports Med.* 2006; 34(3): 407-414.

[24] Smith CD, Slexander S, Hill AM, et al. A biomechanical comparison of single and double-row fixation in arthroscopic rotator cuff repair. *J. Bone Joint Surg. Am.;* 88(11): 2425-2431.

[25] Grimberg J, Diop A, Kalra K, et al. In vitro biomechanical comparison of three different types of single- and double-row arthroscopic rotator cuff repairs: Analysis of continuous bone-tendon contact pressure and surface during different simulated joint positions. *J. Shoulder Elbow Surg.* 2010; 19: 236-243.

[26] Milano G, Grasso A, Zarelli D, et al. Comparison betweeen single-row and double-row rotator cuff repair: a biomechanical study. *Knee Surg. Sports Traumatol. Arthrosc.* 2008; 16(1): 75-80.

[27] Nelson CO, Sileo MJ, Grossman MG, et al.. Single-row modified mason-allen versus double-row arthroscopic rotator cuff repair: a biomechanical and surface area comparison. *Arthroscopy* 2008; 24(8): 941-948.

[28] Brady PC, Arrigoni P, Burkhart SS. Evaluation of residual rotator cuff defects after in vivo single- versus double-row rotator cuff repairs. *Arthroscopy* 2006; 22(10): 1070-1075.

[29] Baums MH, Buchhorn GH, Spahn G, et al. Biomechanical characteristics of single-row repair in comparison to double-row repair

with consideration of the suture configuration and suture material. *Knee Surg. Sports Traumatol. Arthrosc.* 2008; 16(11): 1052-1060.

[30] Charousset C, Grimberg J, Duranthon LD, et al. Can a double-row anchorage technique improve tendn healing in arthroscopic rotator cuff repair?: A prospective, nonrandomized, comparative study of double-row and single-row anchorage techniques with computed tomographic arthrography tendon healing assessment. *Am. J. Sports Med.* 2007; 35(8): 1247-1253.

[31] Franceschi F, Ruzzini L, Longo UG, et al. Equivalent clinical results of arthroscopic single-row and double-row suture anchor repair for rotator cuff tears: a randomized control trial. *Am. J. Sports Med.* 2007; 35(8): 1254-1260.

[32] Park JY, Lhee SH, Choi JH, et al. Comparison of the clinical outcomes of single- and double-row repairs in rotator cuff tears. *Am. J. Sports Med.* 2008; 36(7): 1310-1316.

[33] Grasso A, Milano G, Salvatore M, et al. Single-row versus double-row arthroscopic rotator cuff repair: a prospective randomized clinical study. *Arthroscopy* 2009; 25(1): 4-12.

[34] Burks RT, Crim J, Brown N, et al. A prospective randomized clinical trial comparing arthroscopic single- and double-row rotator cuff repair: magnetic resonance imaging and early clinical evaluation. *Am. J. Sports Med.* 2009; 37(4): 674-682.

[35] Pennington WT, Gibbons DJ, Bartz BA, et al. Comparative analysis of single-row versus double-row repair of rotator cuff tears. *Arthroscopy* 2010; 26(11): 1419-1426.

[36] Trappey GJ, Gartsman GM. *A systematic review of the clinical outcomes of single row versus double row rotator cuff repairs*; 20(2 Suppl): S14-19.

[37] Sher JS, Uribe JW, Posada A et al. Abnormal findings on magnetic resonance images of asymptomatic shoulder. *J. Bone Joint Surg. Am.* 1995; 77: 10-15.

[38] Cordasco FA, Backer M, Craig EV et al. The partial-thickness rotator cuff tear: Is acromioplasty without repair sufficient? *Am. J. Sports Med.* 2002; 30: 257-260.

[39] Ozaki J, Fujimoto S, Nakagawa Y et al. Tears of the rotator cuff of the shoulder associated with pathological changes in cadaver. *J. Bone Joint Surg. Am.* 1988; 70: 1224-1230.

[40] Tamanaka K, Matsumoto T. The joint side of the rotator cuff: A follow-up study by arthrography. *Clin. Orthop. Relat. Res*. 1994; 304: 68-73.

[41] Mazzocca AD, Rincon LM, O'Connor RW, et al. Intra-articular partial-thickness rotator cuff tears: analysis of injured and repaired strain behaviour. *Am. J. Sports Med*. 2008; 36(1): 110-116.

[42] Yang S, Park HS, Flores S, et al. Biomechanical analysis of bursal-sided partial thickness rotator cuff tears. *J. Shoulder Elbow Surg.* 2009;18(3):379-85.

[43] Park JY, Yoo MJ, Kim MH. Comparison of surgical outcome between bursal and articular partial thickness rotator cuff tears. *Orthopedics* 2003; 26(4): 387-390.

[44] Liem D, Alci S, Dedy N et al. Clinical and structural results of partial supraspinatus tears treated by subacromial decompression without repair. *Knee Surg. Sports Traumatol. Arthrosc*. 2008; 16(10): 967-972.

[45] Snyder SJ, Pachelli AF, Del Pizzo W et al. Partial thickness rotator cuff tears: results of arthroscopic treatment. *Arthroscopy* 1991; 7(1): 1-7.

[46] Reynolds SB, Dugas JR, Cain EL, et al. Debridement of small partial-thickness rotator cuff tears in elite overhead throwers. *Clin. Orthop. Relat. Res.* 2008; 466(3): 614-621.

[47] Park JY, Chung KT, Yoo MJ. A serial comparison of arthroscopic repairs for partial- and full-thickness rotator cuff tears. *Arthroscopy* 2004; 20(7): 705-711.

[48] Deutsch A. Arthroscopic repair of partial-thickness tears of the rotator cuff. *J. Shoulder Elbow Surg.* 2007; 16(2): 193-201.

[49] Spencer EE Jr. Partial-thickness articular surface rotator cuff tears: an all-inside repair technique. *Cli. Orthop. Relat. Res*. 2010; 468(6): 1514-1520

[50] Seo YJ, Yoo YS, Kim DY et al. Trans-tendon arthroscopic repair for partial-thickness articular side tears of the rotator cuff. *Knee Surg. Sports Traumatol. Arthrosc. 2011* [Epub ahead of print].

[51] Strauss EJ, Salata MJ, Kercher J et al. The arthroscopic management of partial-thickness rotator cuff tears: a systematic review of the literature. *Arthroscopy* 2011; 27(4): 568-580.

[52] Hirooka A, Yoneda M, Wakaitani S, et al. Augmentation with a Gore-Tex patch for repair of large rotator cuff tears that cannot be sutured. *J. Orthop. Sci.* 2002; 7(4): 451-456.

[53] Encalada-Diaz I, Cole BJ, Macgillivray JD et al. Rotator cuff repair augmentation using a novel polycarbonate polyurethane patch:

Premliminary results at 12 months' follow-up. *J. Shoulder Elbow Surg.* 2010 [Epub ahead of print].

[54] Nada AN, Debnath UK, Robinson DA, et al. Treatment of massive rotator-cuff tears with a polyester ligament (Dacron) augmentation: clinical outcome. *J. Bone Joint Surg. Br.* 2010; 92(10): 1397-1401.

[55] Wong I, Burns J, Snyder S. Arthroscopic GraftJacket repair of rotator cuff tears. *J. Shoulder Elbow Surg.* 2010; 19(2 Suppl): 104-109.

[56] Bond JL, Dopirak RM, Higgins RM et al. Arthroscopic replacement of massive, irreparable rotator cuff tears using a GraftJacket allograft: technique and preliminary results. *Arthroscopy* 2008; 24(4): 403-409.

[57] Burkhead WZ, Schifferen SC, Krishnan SG. Use of Graftjacket as an augmentation for massive rotator cuff tears. *Arthroplasty* 2008; 18(1): 11-18.

[58] Sano H, Mineta M, Kita A, et al. Tendon patch grafting using the long head of the biceps for irreparable massive rotator cuff tears. *J. Orthop. Sci.* 2010; 15(3): 310-316.

[59] Bektaser B, Ocguder A, Solak S et al. Free coracoacromial ligament graft for augmentation of massive rotator cuff tears treated with mini-open repair. *Acta Orthop. Traumatol. Turc.* 2010; 44(6): 426-430.

[60] Mallon WJ, Wilson RJ, Basamania CJ. The association of suprascapular neuropathy with massive rotator cuff tears: a preliminary report. *J. Shoulder Elbow Surg.* 2006;15(4):395-8.

[61] Costouros JG, Porramatikul M, Lie DT. Reversal of suprascapular neuropathy following arthroscopic repair of massive supraspinatus and infraspinatus rotator cuff tears. *Arthroscopy* 2007 Nov;23(11):1152-61.

[62] Randelli PS, Arrigoni P, Cabitza P et al. Autologous platelet rich plasma for arthroscopic rotator cuff repair. A pilot study. *Disabil. Rehabil.* 2008; 30(20-22): 1584-1589.

[63] Randelli P, Arrigoni P, Ragone V et al. Platelet rich plasma in arthroscopic rotator cuff repair: a prospective RCT study, 2-year follow-up. *J. Shoulder Elbow Surg.* 2011; 20(4): 518-528.

[64] Castricini R, Longo UG, De Benedetto M et al. Platelet-rich plasma augmentation for arthroscopic rotator cuff repair: a randomized controlled trial. *Am. J. Sports Med.* 2011; 39(2): 258-265.

[65] Jiang Y, Vaessen B, Lenvik T et al. Multipotent progenitor cells can be isolated from postnatal murine bone marrow, muscle and brain. *Exp. Haematol.* 2002; 30: 896-904.

[66] Mazocca AD, McCarthy MB, Chowaniec DM, et al. Rapid isolation of human stem cells (connective tissue progenitor cells) from the proximal

humerus during arthroscopic rotator cuff surgery. *Am. J. Sports Med.* 2010; 38(7): 1438-1447.

[67] Chang CH, Chen CH, Su CY, et al. Rotator cuff repair with periosteum for enhancing tendon-bone healing: a biomechanical and histological study in rabbits. *Knee Surg. Sports Traumatol. Arthrosc.* 2009; 17(12): 1447-1453.

[68] Gulotta LV, Kovacevic D, Ehteshami JR, et al. Application of bone marrow-derived mesenchymal stem cells in a rotator cuff repair model. *Am. J. Sports Med.* 2009; 37(11): 2126-2133.

[69] Gulotta LV, Kovacevic D, Montgomery S, et al. Stem cells genetically modified with the developmental gene MT1-MMP improve regeneration of the supraspinatus tendon-to-bone insertion site. *Am. J. Sports Med.* 2010; 38(7): 1429-1437.

[70] Hoffmann A, Gross G. Tendon and ligament engineering in the adult organism: mesenchymal stem cells and gene-therapeutic approaches. *Int. Orthop.* 2007; 31: 791-797.

[71] Shahab-Osterloh S, Witte F, Hoffmann A, et al. Mesenchymal sstem cell-dependent formation of heterotopic tendon-bone insertions (Osteotendinous Junctions). *Stem. Cells* 2010; 28: 1590-1601.

[72] Kovacevic D, Rodeo SA. Biological augmentation of rotator cuff tendon repair. *Clin. Orthop. Relat. Res.* 2008; 466: 622-633.

[73] Yao J, Korotkova T, Riboh J, et al. Bioactive sutures for tendon repair: assessment of a method of delivering pluripotential embryonic cells. *J. Hand Surg. Am.* 2008; 33(9): 1558-1564.

[74] Yao J, Korotkova T, Smith RL. Viability and proliferation of pluripotential cells delivered to tendon repair sites using bioactive sutures- an in vitro study. *J. Hand Surg. Am.* 2011; 36(2): 252-258.

In: Arthroscopy
Editors: K. Elani et al.

ISBN: 978-1-61470-955-8
© 2012 Nova Science Publishers, Inc.

Chapter II

Arthroscopy and Stem Cells: Current Treatments and Future Prospects in Orthopaedics

S. B. M. MacLean, J. A. A. Hendriks* and M. Snow

Royal Orthopaedic Hospital NHS Foundation Trust,
Birmingham, United Kingdom

INTRODUCTION

From its infancy in the 1950s onwards [1], arthroscopic instrumentation and technique has evolved exponentially. An increasing number of procedures are performed arthroscopically through the increasing sophistication of surgical equipment and the heightened awareness and education amongst the orthopaedic community. This has led to the arthroscopic treatment of a greater range of joints and pathologies. Compared to conventional open surgical procedures, arthroscopic procedures are less likely to result in complications connected to the necessity for larger incisions. They are less invasive for patients and may result in a lower chance of infection, less postoperative pain

---

* Dr. J.Hendriks is one of the inventors of INSTRUCT and founders of CellCoTec.

and faster repair following surgery. There are obvious benefits to the patient and through better health economics, the whole community.

The possibility of choosing an arthroscopic approach for an operation involving small implants or stem cells is largely limited by the instrumentation required, size of potential implant, fixation technique or other technical complications to deliver the defect proper treatment. Arthroscopic applications demand highly skilled and trained surgeons. To further support training of surgeons in the increasing demands this technology asks, virtual reality training programs are in development [2]. For all new surgical technology in development, other crucial factors to be considered include; potential for clinical success, ease of application for the surgeon, and the required operating room time and cost. A combination of these components influences the adoption rate of the procedure in the medical community as a whole.

Coupled with the advance in arthroscopy has been the development of stem cell research and its application to orthopedic pathology. A fusion of these technologies has led to some studies reporting the successful harvesting of stem cells arthroscopically or the arthroscopic treatment of disease using stem cells.

In this chapter we highlight the opportunities for new technology in current development applying stem cells, and the opportunity or limitations to combine these with an arthroscopic delivery.

POTENTIAL SOURCES OF STEM CELLS

Multipotent stem cells such as mesenchymal cells (MSC's) are generally restricted to a particular germ layer. MSC's are capable of differentiating into bone, cartilage, tendon, ligament and fat – all applicable for use to the Orthopaedic Surgeon. [3] Blood or Bone marrow aspirate (eg the bone marrow of the iliac crest or femur) is a readily accessible source for mesenchymal stem cells (MSC's) and has been used in numerous trials. The initial percentage of MSC's in bone marrow aspirate is approximately 0.1%, however through culturing these cells, a number of MSCs can be obtained, enough for direct arthroscopic implantation for the treatment of disease. MSC's have also been isolated from the periosteum, fat and synovium. [4,5] Transdifferentiation can occur between cell types. Therefore, haematopoietic stem cells may have the potential to from musculoskeletal cells and have reported positive outcomes in fracture repair. [6,7] Drawbacks of using MSC's may include reduced availability with age, [8] the need for culturing before implantation, and cell senescence with loss of multilineage differentiation capability after 34-50 population doublings. [9]

Embryonic stem cells (ESC's) derived from the inner cells of the blastocyst can be used. These have an infinite lifespan and are totipotent. Ethical concerns exist, as does the risk of teratoma formation. More recently, human-induced pluripotent stem cells were generated by the ectopic expression of ESC-specific transcription factors in somatic cells, and although this is a highly specialised technique, may circumvent ethical concerns with ESC's. [10] Foetal stem cells, especially amniotic fluid stem cells (AFS) are a potential source. AFS can be readily obtained through amniocentesis. These cells contain high a high proliferative capacity (>300 population doublings in culture due to preservation of telomere length) and a high differentiation potential. [11]

DELIVERY OF STEM CELLS
THROUGH BIOMATERIALS

Biomaterials can be made of natural materials like hydrogels, or solid biomaterials made of extracellular matrix originating proteins like collagen or hyaluronate. Hydrogels like fibrin can absorb large amounts of water and by regulating their crosslinks their porosity can be changed, allowing encapsulation of cells while its permeability supports cell survival and tissue formation. Natural solid biomaterials have some mechanical properties but because of their limited porosity, cells are seeded onto the surface of these scaffolds. New processing technology, like micro-spinning which does not involve high temperature or aggressive chemical compounds allows the manufacturing of a 3D-porous scaffold with these natural materials. [12]

The synthetic biomaterials applied in regenerative medicine are predominantly based on Poly(α) hydroxyesters such as poly(glycolic acid) (PGA), poly(lactic acid) (PLA) and poly (lactide-co-glycolide acid) (PLGA). The major advantage of these copolymers over natural materials is that they can be tailored to specific applications and provide mechanical properties and lack the disadvantage of the xeno- or allogenic origin of natural biomaterials. [13]

In regenerative medicine a scaffold can be defined as a 3D delivery carrier for cells, growth factors and/or signalling molecules. In addition and depending on the material applied they potentially can provide mechanical stability to the implant site up to comparable levels as the surrounding tissue. Related to this, the necessity to form the biomaterial to mimic the defect's anatomical shape is apparent when treating larger defects. More advanced biomaterials in development aim at regulating the release of growth factors and/or signalling molecules which support tissue regeneration by stem cells either delivered with the scaffold or attracted to the implant site. Physiological events of tissue regeneration or wound healing show that it involves a spatial-, timely- and concentration-dependent delivery of growth factors. Realising a localised delivery of growth factors and/or signalling molecules in a spatio-temporal manner is an ambitious and necessary goal in the way forward for biomaterial-release mechanisms in regenerative medicine [14-15] Finally, depending on the application, a biomaterial scaffold can be either biodegradable-and in time will be replaced by regenerating tissue, or is non-degradable-and will provide enough space to build-up a tissue to regenerate while providing continuous support. [16]

The possibility to apply biomaterials arthroscopically appears to be limited by the specifications of the biomaterial applied and the anticipated necessity to ensure targeted delivery of cells to the defect site. Arthroscopic delivery of a porous scaffold made of solid biomaterial, requires it to be flexible enough to fit through an arthroscope. Alternatively, hydrogel biomaterials allow liquid state scaffold delivery through an arthroscope, to solidify in the defect by means of temperature, pH, infrared or monodisperse two-phase droplet fusion or other. [17-18] New developments in biomaterials making use of biological processes involving proteins and enzymes, would allow arthroscopic or even syringe delivery when they will fill a defect through self assembly. [19]

Finally, the method required to support good fixation of the implant is key in allowing or preventing an arthroscopic procedure. Fixation of constructs for regenerative medicine enhances the need for temporary fixation with biodegradable materials, which disappear whilst new tissue is regenerating in the defect site. [20] Application of numerous sutures to keep constructs, tissue flaps or biomaterials in place are arduous to apply for the surgeon and require an open procedure. Potential candidates are pins, screws or suture anchors, which can be a solid version of the same candidate synthetic biomaterials identified previously for scaffold manufacturing. [21] Alternatively and depending on the anticipated loading and shear forces applied on the implant, it might be sufficient to apply a tissue glue or press fit techniques with which through shaping support a scaffold to stay in place or implanting scaffolds to an appropriate depth not requiring any additional fixation

STEM CELL APPLICATION IN MUSCULOSKELETAL INJURY AND DISEASE – WHERE ARE WE NOW?

Bone

A fracture in a healthy host, with healthy bone and surrounding tissue normally provides enough inflammatory response with cytokine migration and angiogenic growth factors to ensure an adequate environment for bone healing. Fractures leading to significant bone loss require replacement of bone to ensure structural integrity, healing and ultimately limb function. Tumour resection, revision surgery, developmental deformities and infection can lead to significant bone loss and poor potential for healing. Traditional strategies include vascularised bone grafting, distraction osteogenesis, autologous and allograft bone grafting and demineralised bone grafting. These methods are often technically challenging and all have their potential disadvantages. [22]

Successful regeneration of bone usually requires osteoproduction, osteoinduction, osteoconduction and mechanical stimulation. Therefore, osteogenic cells, a scaffold, growth factors, suitable microenvironment, the correct mechanical stress and strain ideally are needed as well as blood vessels and a nutrient supply. [22] There have been trials in rats [23], dogs [24] and several human trials thus far. [25] Debate arises as to the optimal delivery of the stem cells to the defective tissue. Dupont et al [26] recently showed in rats that both MSC's and foetal stem cells when delivered to a fracture site resulted in significantly enhanced bone growth compared to controls. The stem cells also 'targeted' the contralateral bone defect.

MSC's have been used for the generation of fully-vascularised bone flaps of the desired shape. During these procedures, MSC's are loaded into appropriate carriers and transplanted into a non-skeletal site surrounding an artery or vein. The vascularised bone-flap is grown, then transported into the target bone defect. This has shown some success in animal models. Kamei et al has shown the ability to grow bone in the omentum of rabbits using this technique. [27]

Early stages of avascular necrosis in the femoral heads of humans have been treated with autologous bone marrow implantation with some success as compared to traditional treatments such as core decompression. Unfortunately these studies are limited by small numbers in each treatment arm. [28] Percutaneous implantation of these cells has been shown to lead to a significant improvement in pain and function. [29] Further better-quality evidence is needed to determine the success of this treatment.

Osteogenesis imperfecta (OI) is a genetic disease causing defective production of type 1 collagen. This usually results in pathological fractures causing severe morbidity. Studies have shown that intrauterine transplantation of human blood foetal stem/stromal cells in mice with osteogenesis imperfect resulted in a significant reduction of bone fracture. Other studies have shown that MSC's infused into irradiated mice with OI produced normal bone concentrations of type 1 collagen. [30] Future studies are needed to look at the therapeutic benefit of these interventions in humans.

As already explained, a number of extracellular factors are critical for the regeneration of bone. It is likely that MSC's and other mononucleated cells contribute directly to bone repair but also enhance repair through the secretion of paracrine factors and cell-to-cell contact. The use of an appropriate scaffold is also vital. Cuomo [31] recently showed in rats that the use of a MSC-enriched aspirate did not enhance osteogenesis as compared to normal bone marrow aspirate control. In his model, demineralised bone matrix was used which may not have provided cell-signalling potential to lead to repair. When rhBMP-2 was added there was a 100% bone-healing rate. The micro-structure of the scaffold may also be important. Graziano [32] showed that superior bone formation occurred in scaffolds with microcavities, which enhanced cell adhesion compared to smooth scaffolds.

Longitudinal fractures through the physis in children often causes bony bridges to develop resulting in shortening or an angular deformity. Surgical options in older children includes stapling, epiphyseodesis, and osteotomy. Treatment is more limited in younger children. Ahn et al [33] showed that MSC's in 10% gelatine in Gelfoam with TGF-β^3 markedly reduced angular deformity after partial physeal defects in rabbits. In these instances, the addition of growth factor provides an appropriate external signal for chondrogenic differentiation. Lee et al [34] found that implantation of MSC's into growth-plate defects resulted in a significant reduction in growth arrest in the rabbit tibia.

As yet no marker has been identified for osteogenic differentiation of adult stem cells. A marker is vital to ensure that the implanted stem cells being used are differentiating and contributing to bone regeneration.

Cartilage

Articular cartilage is generally regarded a post-mitotic tissue. It is a uniquely avascular, aneural and alymphatic load-bearing tissue that is supported by the underlying subchondral bone plate. Traditionally it was thought of that cartilage consisted of terminally differentiated cells. Recent studies however have challenged this view. Articular cartilage has been found to demonstrate a distinct pattern regarding stem cell markers (Notch-1, Stro-1, and VCAM-1) [35], and there has been a positive identification of side population cells in articular cartilage. [36]This supports the theory that articular cartilage has residing stem cells.

Articular cartilage has a limited potential to heal. Cartilage defects may cause pain, swelling, locking and eventually lead to osteoarthritis. There is of yet, no universally agreed gold standard for treatment. [37]

Combination Treatments Involving Cartilage and Stem Cells

In cartilage repair, common applications for stem cells applied arthroscopically are Microfracture and Autologous Cartilage Implantation (ACI). With microfracture, bone marrow from the underlying bone is allowed to enter the defect site by penetrating the subchondral bone. Microfracture is applied in clinical studies and practised in several orthopaedic area's; knee [38], hip [39], ankle [40] and shoulder [41-42]. Traditionally the repair of cartilage seems to be limited to the formation of fibrocartilage (predominately disorganised type 1 collagen) resulting in poor mechanical properties compared to that of hyaline cartilage. Microfracture has traditionally been accepted as a good first line treatment leading to short term alleviation of symptoms limited by defect size and well contained lesions in young patients.

From the findings of microfracture studies, one can conclude that the stem cells in the bone marrow penetrating from the subchondral bone are not sufficient to support long-term cartilage repair. This can be caused by two factors; firstly the limited number of stem cells in bone marrow (< 0.1%) is insufficient to initiate a satisfactory repair reaction. Secondly, additional support to lead to a satisfactory cartilage repair reaction is required for the limited number of stem cells in the bone marrow to regenerate cartilage. The potential contribution of heterogenic cells in the bone marrow called mononucleated cells to tissue repair is important. [43]

The limited number of stem cells in bone marrow can be circumvented by isolating stem cells from bone marrow and expansion in vitro. This inevitably leads to a chance of phenotypically changing the cells during the culturing process. It is unclear how this influences the contribution of stem cells to a regenerative tissue repair reaction upon implantation. In addition, this will complicate the process leading to a two-stage procedure with 3-5 weeks between operations, similarly as ACI, leading to the same disadvantages as outlined later in the chapter.

This additional support for stem cells or mononucleated cells in the bone marrow to contribute to a tissue repair reaction might come from biomaterials which provide the cells with cues through their material and/or surface properties, growth factors, extracellular proteins or any combination of these three.

Autologous chondrocyte implantation (ACI) – combines chondrocytes with stem cells from the periosteum, which is sutured over the defect site for chondral defects, or in addition with stem cells from penetrating bone marrow when applied to osteochondral defects. The resulting cartilage contains a mixed hyaline/fibrocartilage type repair tissue containing abundant levels of type 2 collagen. This has been correlated to long-term clinical benefits. [44] ACI, however, is a two step procedure requiring an initial arthroscopic surgery to take a cartilage biopsy and a second procedure 3-5 weeks later to implant the cells. Implantation is performed by an open procedure to allow application of a substantial amount of sutures to secure the periosteum above the defect site, inject the cells under the periosteum and keep the cells in place under the periosteum with fibrin glue. Even though clinically several publications showed its long-term benefits in patient outcome and tissue repair [44], it is generally conceived as a complicated surgical procedure by the orthopaedic community and because of it complexity appears to have limited health economic benefits [45, 46] preventing it to reach many patients with cartilage defects in need for treatment but not yet ready for a total joint replacement.

Stem cells or chondrocyte pre-cursors can be applied to aid cartilage repair. Hui et al [47] showed that chondrocytes and MSC's had comparable enhancing effects on the repair of chondral defects in advanced osteochondritis dissecans, both of which were superior to mosaicoplasty (osteochondral autograft from a non-weight bearing area) and periosteal graft usage. Ten year follow-up after ACI has shown that with good patient selection, the majority of patients may continue to have good symptom relief, despite a high re-operation rate [48]. There is some evidence that patients may benefit at longer-term follow-up. The use of mature articular chondrocytes however, is restricted in that it is limited by cell senescence, and expansion in culture may induce de-differentiation. [49]

New developments in cartilage repair which combine cells with a biomaterial, aim to realize a single stage procedure by cartilage autograft implantation system (CAIS) applying minced-up cartilage reinforced with fibrin glue onto a polydioxanone-reinforced foam [46] or cellular cartilage instruction technology (INSTRUCT) which combines primary freshly isolated chondrocytes with mononucleated cells from bone marrow seeded into a 3D deposited porous PEGT/PBT scaffold. In a preclinical study, 12 month results in horses show arthroscopic, histologic, and immunohistochemistry results to be superior to both implantation techniques tested (ACI and CAIS) compared with empty defects and defects with polydioxanone foam alone [46] . Initial clinical results for the CAIS approach at 2 years show it's a safe procedure and generates significantly better patient quality of life scores compared to microfracture, while no significant difference was shown in defect filling and integration at this follow-up time [45].

Preclinical results of a combination of primary chondrocytes with bone marrow cells in publications from several authors showed that the cellular interaction between the two cell types support cartilage tissue formation while preventing hypertrophic differentiation of the bone marrow cells [44, 50-52]. In addition, preclinical results of INSTRUCT, for which the cell combination was established during a single surgical procedure, show that it appears to exceed the previously identified clinical benefits of ACI in an immune deficient mouse model applying human cells. The nude mice model was identified as the most relevant and predictive for clinical efficacy by the highest quality clinical study in cartilage repair performed so far [44]. Therein, the clinical outcome at 3 yr follow-up has been demonstrated to correlate with cell markers assessed before cell implantation [53], which have been setup to correlate with nude mice cartilage formation data.

Both approaches, INSTRUCT and CAIS are still in clinical investigation to prove their safety and support long-term solutions for cartilage repair. The combination of a single stage procedure providing cells and a scaffold which provides a simple delivery system and mechanical support immediately after implantation (INSTRUCT), would lead to increased patient benefit and improved health economics as a whole.

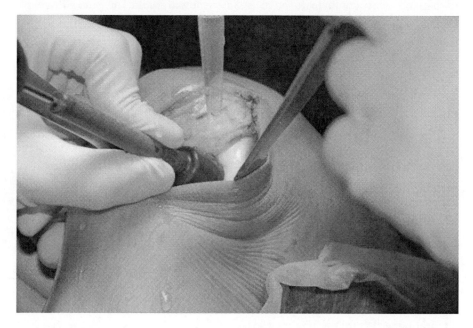

Measurement of the defect size prior to application of the cell/scaffold implant.

Delivery methods of MCS for cartilaginous defects have been studied. There are obvious potential surgical complications in performing arthrotomy for repairing cartilaginous defects in the knee, such as infection, wound problems, and weakness in the extensor mechanism or anterior knee pain, for instance. Kobayashi showed that an external magnetic device under arthroscopic control could be used to deliver magnetically-labelled MSC's to an osteochondral defect of the patella. [54] Although there were limitations to the study and the chondrogenic-affecting potential of the ferumoxides used in the study is debatable, it demonstrates a novel approach to the targeted delivery of stem cells.

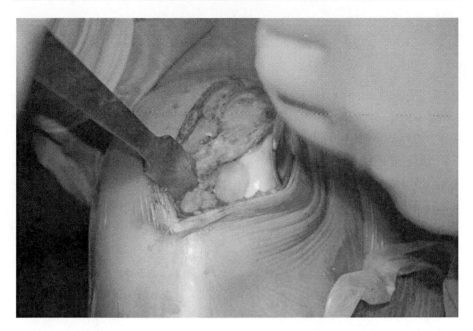

The knee chondral defect debrided with the cell/scaffold implant in place.

Tendons and Ligaments

Tendon and ligaments are often affected by mechanical injuries or chronic impairment and possess a low healing capacity. Autografts, allografts, biomaterials and direct repair have been the traditional options of reconstruction. There are obvious problems with biological grafts include donor site morbidity, lack of available donor material, tissue rejection, and infection. [55]

Experimental studies in animals have been encouraging, using MSC's. Young et al [56] seeded MSC on to a biodegradable scaffold in a 1cm defect in a rabbit Achilles tendon, showing the regeneration of tendinous tissue. Awad showed similar results in the patellar tendon. [57] Smith et al [58] has shown positive benefits in horses – when implanting MSC's in flexor tendon injuries, with ultrasonographic evidence showing no deleterious effect to the tendon and no evidence of heterotopic bone formation.

An important element in the success following anterior cruciate ligament reconstruction (ACL) is the incorporation of the graft to the bony tunnels in the tibia and femur in which it is placed during surgery. The normal anatomy of the insertion site of the ACL is fibrocartilaginous and consists of four distinct zones: ligament substance, unmineralised fibrocartilage, mineralised fibrocartilage and bone. [59] It is difficult to restore this anatomy within six months of surgery, which can lead to early failure of the graft. Lim et al [60] showed that the application of MSC's to tendon grafts at the tendon-bone junction in rabbits results in a zone of fibrocartilage more closely resembling that of the normal ACL; having significant increase in load to failure and stiffness in the first eight weeks after reconstruction of the ACL.

The use of MSC's at osteotendinous junctions has been studied. A recent study illustrates the ability of a sample of MSC's to exhibit osteogenic and tenogenic potential. [61] The study, using rats showed that the process was primarily governed by growth factors and signalling mediators (Smad8 and BMP2) but further shaped by mechanical loading. It has also been shown that the orientation of a fibrous scaffold used with MSC's can influence the differentiation of cell type. Yin et al [62] showed that a randomly-orientated fibrous scaffold induced osteogenesis, while the aligned scaffold hindered the process. Ruptures at osteotendinous junctions are often difficult to repair surgically and healing through fibrosis gives inferior functional performance. MSC's in this context could significantly improve patient outcome.

The supraspinatus tendon on the footprint of the greater tuberosity is a common site for tendinopathy and rupture. A recent study biopsied the supraspinatus tendon, showing that the perivascular cells in this region exhibited tendon and mesenchymal stem cell-like characteristics. The perivascular cells in the tendon may therefore be considered a source for tendon precursor cells, which may give rise to a new generation of tendon cells with internal or external stimulation. [63] Further studies are needed to develop methods to regenerate tendons in areas such as the supraspinatus footprint, exploiting the use of these cell precursors.

Menisci

Meniscal tears in the avascular inner third do not heal spontaneously. Meniscectomy and removal of as little as 15-34% can increase contact pressures between the tibia and femur of 350%, which can lead to early osteoarthritis. [64] Pabbruwe et al [65] recently showed that a new stem cell/collagen scaffold can be used with inner third tears. In the ovine meniscus, analysis showed greater integration of the scaffold compared to cell-free controls. This resulted in an increased tensile strength in the meniscus. Interestingly the addition of TGF-β1 inhibited integration. Other studies using stem cells show similar findings. [66]

Spine

Pre-ganglionic brachial plexus injuries represent the majority of lesions in brachial plexus injuries and carry the worst prognosis. The term implies that the root or rootlet has been avulsed from the spinal cord. These are generally regarded as irreparable. [67] However, evidence of axonal regeneration and functional recovery has been found in animal models using stem cells. Akiyama et al [68] has shown that MSC's isolated in culture can remyelinate demyelinated spinal cord axons after direct injection into the lesion. Gene therapy strategies such as viral-vector mediated gene transfer and intramedullary injections have been proposed.

Degenerative intervertebral disc disease is a common cause of back pain, which is a leading cause of morbidity and is of huge socio-economic cost to society. [69] Approximately 90% of pain settles with conservative measure initially but is often recurrent. Traditional surgical treatment options include discectomy (micro- vs open) +/- fusion. Crevensten et al [70] explored the use of MSC's for intervertebral disc regeneration in rats. MSC's were injected using a 15% hyaluronan gel carrier. A trend towards increased disc height was noticed suggesting an increase in proteoglycan matrix synthesis.

Spinal fusion using autologous bone graft has a significant risk of non-union. [55] Successful stem-cell based fusion has been shown in several studies. [71] Sheyn et al showed that in mice that the distribution of stiffness in an MSC-based fusion group was similar to that in a steel pin fusion group. [72] The morbidity following spinal surgical instrumentation can be high, and stem-cell mediated fusion may obviate these problems.

Skeletal Muscle

Loss of skeletal muscle through trauma, tumour ablation or prolonged denervation are common clinical challenges. Skeletal tissue consists of highly orientated muscle fibres in an extracellular 3D matrix. In studies, nanofibre matrices with parallel alignment has provided an ideal scaffold for cultivating myoblasts. [73] Most work thus far has been on the use of satellite cells-undifferentiated cells which reside between the sarcolemma and the basement membrane, which are committed to the myocyte lineage and can regenerate large parts of damaged muscle in-vivo. In-vitro studies however, have shown that these cells rapidly de-differentiate. Gussoni et al [74] showed that satellite cells transplanted into patients with Duchenne muscular dystrophy retained only 10% of these myoblasts at 6 months. Further studies should look to see whether transplantation of MSC's *and* satellite cells can augment a paracrine effect on cell differentiation therefore muscle regeneration. [75]

SUMMARY

Stem cell therapy holds great potential for musculoskeletal injury and disease. Vital factors in the microenvironment interact including; transplanted growth factors, cell signalling, gene therapy, scaffold structure, as well as the patient's own supply of stem cells, nutrients and blood flow to the target area. The evolving technology in arthroscopic surgery holds hope for arthroscopic application of stem cells to treat orthopaedic pathology in the near future. The orthopaedic community looks forward to future promising research in these areas.

REFERENCES

1. Hurter E. Arthroscopy; a new method of knee examination, *Rev. Chir. Orthop. Reparatrice Appar Mot.* 1955;41(5-6):763-766.
2. Mabrey JD, Reinig KD, Cannon WD. Virtual reality in orthopaedics: is it a reality? *Clin. Orthop. Relat. Res.* 2010 Oct;468(10):2586-91.
3. Caplan AL. The mesengenic process. *Clin. Plast. Surg.* 1994; 21: 429-435.
4. Cenni E, Perut F, Baglio S et al. Recent highlights on bone stem cells: a report from Bone Stem Cells 2009, and not only... *J. Cell Mol. Med.* 2010; 14(11): 2614-2621.
5. Kadiyala S, Jaiswal N, Bruder SP. Culture-expanded, bone marrow-derived mesenchymal stem cells regenerate a critical-sized segmental bone defect. *Tissue Eng.* 1997; 3: 173-185.

6. Bruder SP, Kurth AA, Shea M et al. Bone regeneration by implantation of purified, culture-expanded human mesenchymal stem cells. *J. Orthop. Res.* 1998; 16: 155-162.
7. Caplan AL. *Mesenchymal stem cells in Handbook of Stem Cells 2004.* (Elsevier Academic, New York), Vol 2: pp 299-308.
8. Derubeis AR, Cancedda R. Bone marrow stromal cells (BMSCs) in bone engineering: limitations and recent advances. *Ann. Biomed. Eng.* 2004. 32: 160-165.
9. Bossolasco P, Montemurro T, Cova L et al. Molecular and phenotypic characterisation of human amniotic fluid cells and their differentiation potential. *Cell Res.* 2006; 16: 329-336.
10. Takahashi K, Tanabe K, Ohnuki M et al. Induction of pluripotent sten cells from adult human fibroblasts by defined factors. *Cell* 2007; 131: 861-872.
11. De Coppi P, Pozzobon M, Piccoli M et al. Isolation of mesenchymal stem cells from human vermiform appendix. *J. Surg. Res.* 2006 Sep;135(1):85-91.
12. Jeong SI, Krebs MD, Bonino CA et al. Electrospun chitosan-alginate nanofibers with in situ polyelectrolyte complexation for use as tissue engineering scaffolds. *Tissue Eng. Part A.* 2011 Jan;17(1-2):59-70.
13. Gunja NJ, Athanasiou KA. Biodegradable materials in arthroscopy. *Sports Med. Arthrosc.* 2006 Sep;14(3):112-9.
14. Chen FM, Zhang M, Wu ZF. Toward delivery of multiple growth factors in tissue engineering. *Biomaterials.* 2010; 31(24):6279-308.
15. Guldberg RE. Spatiotemporal delivery strategies for promoting musculoskeletal tissue regeneration. *J. Bone Miner Res.* 2009; 24(9):1507-11.
16. Ahmed TA, Dare EV, Hincke M. Fibrin: a versatile scaffold for tissue engineering applications. *Tissue Eng. Part B Rev.* 2008;14(2):199-215.
17. Cheng YH, Yang SH, Su WY et al. Thermosensitive chitosan-gelatin-glycerol phosphate hydrogels as a cell carrier for nucleus pulposus regeneration: an in vitro study. *Tissue Eng. Part A.* 2010;16(2):695-703.
18. Ziemecka I, Van Steijn V, Koper GJ et al. Monodisperse hydrogel microspheres by forced droplet formation in aqueous two-phase systems. *Lab. Chip.* 2011;11(4):620-4.

19. Hong JS, Stavis SM, DePaoli Lacerda SH et al. Microfluidic directed self-assembly of liposome-hydrogel hybrid nanoparticles. *Langmuir* 2010; 26(13):11581-8.
20. Burkhart SS. The evolution of clinical applications of biodegradable implants in arthroscopic surgery. *Biomaterials*. 2000; 21(24):2631-4.
21. Herbort M, Zelle S, Rosenbaum D, Osada N, Raschke M, Petersen W, Zantop T Arthroscopic fixation of matrix-associated autologous chondrocyte implantation: importance of fixation pin angle on joint compression forces. *Arthroscopy.* 2011; 27(6): 809-16.
22. Pneumaticos SG, Triantafyllopoulos GK, Basdra EK et al. Segmental bone defects: from cellular and molecular pathways to the development of novel biological treatments. *J. Cell Mol. Med.* 2010; 14(11): 2561-2569.
23. Khosla S, Westendorf JJ, Modder UL. Concise Review: Insights from Normal Bone Remodelling and Stem Cell-Based Therapies for Bone Repair. *Stem Cells* 2010; 28: 2124-2128.
24. Bruder SP, Kurth AA, Shea M et al. Bone regeneration by implantation of purified, culture-expanded human mesenchymal stem cells. *J. Orthop. Res.* 1998; 16: 155-162.
25. Bruder SP, Kraus KH, Goldberg VM et al. The effect of implants loaded with autologous mmesennchymal stem cells on the healing of canine segmental bone defects. *J. Bone Joint Surg. Am*. 1998; 80: 985-996.
26. Dupont KM, Sharma K, Stevens HY et al. Human stem cell delivery for treatment of large segmental bone defects. *Proc. Natl. Acad. Sci. USA.* 2010;107(8):3305-10.
27. Kamei Y, Toriyama K, Takada T et al. Tissue-engineering bone from omentum. *Nagoya J. Med. Sci*. 2010;72(3-4):111-7.
28. Gangji V, Hauzeur JP. Treatment of osteonecrosis of the femoral head with implantation of autologous bone-marrow cells. Surgical technique. *J. Bone Joint Surg. Am*. 2005; 87 Suppl 1(Pt 1): 106-12.
29. Yan ZQ, Chen YS, Li WJ. Treatment of osteonecrosis of the femoral head by percutaneous decompression and autologous bone marrow mononuclear cell infusion. *Chin. J. Traumatol.* 2006; 9(1): 3-7.
30. Pereira RF, O'Hara MD, Laptex AV et al. Marrow stromal cells as a source of progenitor cells for nonhaematopoietic tissues in transgenic mice with a phenotype of osteogenesis imperfecta. *Proc. Matl. Acad. Sci. USA* 1998; 95: 1142-1147.

31. Cuomo AV, Virk M, Petrigliano F et al. Menechymal stem cell concentration and bone repair: potential pitfalls from bench to bedside. *J. Bone Joint Surg. Am.* 2009; 91: 1073-1083.

32. Graziano A, D'Aquino R, Cusella-De Angelis MG et al. Concave pit-containing scaffold surfaces improve stem cell-derived osteoblast performance and lead to significant bone tissue formation. *PLoS One;* 2(6):e496.

33. Ahn JI, Canale ST, Butler SD et al. Stem cell repair of physeal cartilage. *J. Orthop. Res.* 2004; 6:1215-21.

34. Lee EH, Chen F, Chan J et al. Treatment of growth arrest by transfer of cultured chondrocytes into physeal defects. *J. Pediatr. Orthop.* 1998; 18(2):155-60.

35. Grogan SP, Miyaki S, Asahara H et al. Mesenchymal progenitor cell markers in human articular cartilage: notmal distribution and changes in osteoarthritis. *Arthritis. Res. Ther.* 2009; 11: R85

36. Dowthwaite GP, Bishop JC, Redman SN et al. The surface of articular cartilage contains a progenitor cell population. *J. Cell Sci.* 2004; 117(6): 889-897.

37. Hunziker EB. Articular cartilage repair: basic science and clinical progress; a review of the current status and prospects. *Osteoarthritis Cartilage* 2002; 10: 432-463.

38. Saris DB, Vanlauwe J, Victor J et al. Characterized chondrocyte implantation results in better structural repair when treating symptomatic cartilage defects of the knee in a randomized controlled trial versus microfracture. *Am. J. Sports Med.* 2008;36(2): 235-46.

39. Yen YM, Kocher MS. Chondral lesions of the hip: microfracture and chondroplasty. *Sports Med. Arthrosc.* 2010;18(2): 83-9.

40. Jung HG, Carag JA, Park JY et al. Role of arthroscopic microfracture for cystic type osteochondral lesions of the talus with radiographic enhanced MRI support. *Knee Surg. Sports Traumatol. Arthrosc.* 2011;19(5): 858-62.

41. Snow M, Funk L. Microfracture of chondral lesions of the glenohumeral joint. *Int. J. Shoulder Surg.* 2008; 2(4):72-6.

42. Elser F, Braun S, Dewing CB et al. Glenohumeral joint preservation: current options for managing articular cartilage lesions in young, active patients. *Arthroscopy* 2010; 26(5): 685-696.

43. Williams R, Khan IM, Richardson K et al. Identification and clonal characterisation of a progenitor cell sub-population in normal human articular cartilage. *PLoS One.* 2010; 5(10): e13246.

44. Saris DB, Vanlauwe J, Victor J et al. Treatment of symptomatic cartilage defects of the knee: characterized chondrocyte implantation results in better clinical outcome at 36 months in a randomized trial compared to microfracture. *Am. J. Sports Med*. 2009;37 Suppl 1:10S-19S.

45. Clar C, Cummins E, McIntyre L. Clinical and cost-effectiveness of autologous chondrocyte implantation for cartilage defects in knee joints: systematic review and economic evaluation. *Health Technol. Assess* 2005;9(47): 1-82.

46. Derrett S, Stokes EA, James M. Cost and health status analysis after autologous chondrocyte implantation and mosaicplasty: a retrospective comparison. *Int. J. Technol. Assess Health Care* 2005; 21(3): 359-67.

47. Hui JH, Chen F, Thambyah A et al. Treatment of chondral lesions in advanced osteochondritis dissecans: a comparative study of the efficacy of chondrocytes, mesenchymal stem cells, periosteal graft, and mosaicoplasty (osteochondral autograft) in animal models. *J. Pediatr. Orthop*. 2004; 24: 427-433.

48. Moseley JB Jr, Anderson AF, Browne JE et al. Long-term durability of autologous chondrocyte implantation: a multicenter, observational study in US patients. *Am. J. Sports Med*. 2010; 38(2): 238-46.

49. Peterson L, Vasiliadis HS, Brittberg M et al. Autologous chondrocyte implantation: a long-term follow-up. *Am. J. Sports Med*. 2010; 38(6): 1117-24.

50. Dai J, Wang X, Shen G. Cotransplantation of autologous bone marrow stromal cells and chondrocytes as a novel therapy for reconstruction of condylar cartilage. *Med. Hypotheses* 2011; 77(1):132-3.

51. Wu L, Leijten JC, Georgi N et al. Trophic effects of mesenchymal stem cells increase chondrocyte proliferation and matrix formation. *Tissue Eng. Part A* 2011;17(9-10):1425-36.

52. Bian L, Zhai DY, Mauck RL et al. Coculture of human mesenchymal stem cells and articular chondrocytes reduces hypertrophy and enhances functional properties of engineered cartilage. *Tissue Eng. Part A* 2011;17(7-8): 1137-45.

53. Dell'Accio F, De Bari C, Luyten FP. Molecular markers predictive of the capacity of expanded human articular chondrocytes to form stable cartilage in vivo. *Arthritis. Rheum*. 2001; 44(7): 1608-19.

54. Hori J, Deie M, Kobayashi T et al. Articular cartilage repair using an intra-articular magnet and synovium-derived cells. *J. Orthop. Res.* 2011; 29(4): 531-8.

55. Lee EH, Hui JHP. The potential of stem cells in orthopaedic surgery. *J. Bone Joint Surg. Br.* 2006; 88(7): 841-51.

56. Young RG, Butler DL, Weber W et al. Use of mesenchymal stem cells in a collagen matrix for Achilles tendon repair. *J. Orthop. Res.* 1998;16(4): 406-13.

57. Awad HA, Boivin GP, Dressler MR et al. Repair of patellar tendon injuries using a cell-collagen composite. *J. Orthop. Res.* 200;21(3): 420-31.

58. Smith RK. Mesenchymal stem cell therapy for equine tendinopathy. *Disabil. Rehabil.* 2008; 30(20-22): 1752-8.

59. Hyman J, Rodeo SA. Injury and repair of tendons and ligaments. *Phys. Med. Rehabil. Clin. N. Am.* 2000; 11: 267-288.

60. Lim JK, Hui J, Li L, Thambyah A, Goh J, Lee EH. Enhancement of tendon graft osteointegration using mesenchymal stem cells in a rabbit model of anterior cruciate ligament reconstruction. *Arthroscopy.* 2004; 20(9): 899-910.

61. Shahab-Osterloh S, Witte F, Hoffmann A. Mesenchymal stem cell-dependent formation of heterotopic tendon-bone insertions (osteotendinous junctions). *Stem Cells* 2010; 28(9): 1590-601.

62. Yin Z, Chen X, Chen JL et al. The regulation of tendon stem cell differentiation by the alignment of nanofibers. *Biomaterials.* 2010; 31(8): 2163-75.

63. Tempfer H, Wagner A, Gehwolf R. Perivascular cells of the supraspinatus tendon express both tendon- and stem cell-related markers. *Histochem. Cell Biol.* 2009; 131(6): 733-741.

64. Allen PR, Denham RA, Swan AV. Late degenerative changes after meniscectomy: factors affecting the knee after operation. *J. Bone Joint Surg. Br.* 1984; 66-B: 666-671.

65. Pabbruwe MB, Kafienah W, Tarlton. Repair of meniscal cartilage white zone tears using a stem cell/collagen-scaffold implant. *Biomaterials.* 2010; 31(9): 2583-91.

66. Dutton A, Hui JPP, Lee EH et al. Enhancement of meniscal repair using mesenchymal stem cells ina porcine model. *Procs 5th Combined Meeting of the Orthopaedic Research Societies of USA, Canada, Japan and Europe, 2004.*

67. Chuang DC. Adult brachial plexus reconstruction with the level of injury: review and personal experience. *Plast. Reconstr. Surg.* 2009; 124(6 Suppl):e359-69.

68. Akiyama Y, Radtke C, Kocsis JD. Remyelination of the rat spinal cord by transplantation of identified bone marrow stromal cells. *J. Neurosci.* 2002; 22(15): 6623-30.

69. Maclean S, Chambers C, Clarke A. Chapter 5-Back Pain In: *Clarke A (Ed) et al ABC of Spinal Disorders.* West Sussex, UK. Blackwell Publishing Ltd. 2010: pp 19-21.

70. Crevensten G, Walsh AJ, Ananthaktishnan D et al. Intervertebral disc cell therapy for regeneration: mesenchymal stem cell implantation in rat intervertebral discs. *Ann. Biomed. Eng.* 2004; 32: 430-434.

71. Steinmann JC, Herkowitz HN. Pseudoarthrosis of the spine. *Clin. Orthop.* 1992; 284: 80-90.

72. Sheyn D, Rüthemann M, Mizrahi O et al. Genetically modified mesenchymal stem cells induce mechanically stable posterior spine fusion. *Tissue Eng. Part A.* 2010; 16(12): 3679-86.

73. Huang NF, Patel S, Thakar RG et al. Myotube assembly on nanofibrous and micropatterned polymers, *Nano Lett.* 2006; 6: 537-542.

74. Gussoni E, Blau HM, Kunkel LM. The fate of individual myoblasts after transplantation into muscles of DMD patients. *Nat. Med.* 1997; 3(9): 970-7.

75. Klumpp D, Horch RE, Knesner U et al. Engineering sskeletal muscle tissue-new perspectives in vitro and in vivo. *J. Cell Mol. Med.* 2010; 14(11): 2622-2629.

In: Arthroscopy

ISBN: 978-1-61470-955-8

Editors: K. Elani et al.

© 2012 Nova Science Publishers, Inc.

Chapter III

Hip Arthroscopy: Indications, Technique and Future Perspectives

*E. A. Audenaert,[1] C. A. Pattyn,[1] H. Budd,[2] and V. Khanduja[2]**

[1]Ghent University Hospital, Ghent, Belgium
[2]Addenbrooke's Cambridge University Hospital, Cambridge, United Kingdom

ABSTRACT

Hip arthroscopy has evolved from an experimental and mainly diagnostic tool, to a standard and effective surgical procedure for the diagnosis and treatment of a variety of disorders not only within but outside the hip as well. The procedure allows for a less invasive approach leading to a faster recovery and decreased peri-operative morbidity compared with the alternative approach of exposing the joint via surgical dislocation of the hip. Furthermore, the recent discovery of Femoroacetabular impingement (FAI) coupled with the surge of interest

* Corresponding Author: Mr. Vikas Khanduja MBBS, MRCS (G), MSc, FRCS, FRCS (Orth), Consultant Orthopaedic Surgeon, Addenbrooke's – Cambridge University Hospitals, Box 37, Hills Road, Cambridge CB2 0QQ, United Kingdom. Tel: 44 1223 309524. Email: vk29@cam.ac.uk.

in sports surgery around the hip has led to improvement of techniques in clinical examination around the hip and imaging as well. This has meant that conditions which were previously unrecognized are being described and can be effectively treated with hip arthroscopy. However, the procedure has a long learning curve, requires appropriate training and specialized equipment and is not for the occasional operator. The results of surgery are dependent on careful patient selection and meticulous pre-operative planning.

The aim of this chapter, therefore, is present to the reader a systematic approach to history, clinical examination and investigations of a young adult with hip pain, a detailed account of the technical aspects of hip arthroscopy, the indications for which it is useful along with the possible complications and contraindications. Finally, a brief description of the current research in our departments and future developments of this exciting procedure will be discussed.

APPROACH TO A YOUNG ADULT WITH HIP PAIN

Assessment of a young adult with hip pain commences with a precise history and careful examination to determine the presence of surgically treatable intra-articular or extra-articular pathology.

History

A structured history should include the patients age, occupation, recreational interests and expectations and elicit the nature, severity and onset of symptoms including pain, clicking, locking, stiffness, instability and longevity (Table 1). A number of patients may present with prolonged symptoms in which case it is crucial to isolate those that are acute, mechanical and may respond to surgery from the chronic symptoms typically relating to chondral damage and offer a less predictable surgical outcome[1]. Those with mechanical symptoms including sharp stabbing pain, clicking and locking are more likely to respond to hip arthroscopy than patients with aching pain independent of activity [1]. The presence of groin pain and radiation to the medial thigh relates to the principle innervator of the hip being the L3 nerve root, which provides sensory innervation to this cutaneous area [2].

Table 1. Structured History

Location of pain (groin, lateral, posterior)
Severity of pain (mild, moderate, severe)
Onset of pain (acute, insidious, relationship to trauma)
Longevity of pain
Exacerbating and relieving factors (activity associated, night pain, constant/intermittent, position of hip associated with onset)
Mechanical symptoms (locking, clicking, sharp stabbing pains)
Effect on activities of daily living, work and recreation
Patient expectations
Previous musculoskeletal history

Isolated posterior hip pain is unusually secondary to underlying hip pathology and caution should be used when considering such a patient for arthroscopy [2,3]. A patient that presents with the classical C-sign, where the hand clasps the lateral hip with thumb on the posterior aspect of the greater trochanter and fingers resting on the groin, is indicative of underlying hip pathology [2]. (Figure 1-A) In a retrospective review of 66 patients with arthroscopically confirmed labrum tears pre-operative symptoms and examination findings were reviewed [3]. This revealed that 92% had groin pain, 86% sharp pain, 91% activity related pain and 95% had a positive impingement test while only 30% reported acute onset pain and as few as 9% related it to a major traumatic episode though it is unclear which patients had the best results, what determined patient selection for hip arthroscopy and who had contiguous chondral lesions. In a larger group of 301 patients undergoing arthroscopic osteoplasty for femoroacetabular impingement the prevalence of groin pain was lower (81%) but the impingement test was positive in 99% of the cases and the FABER test was positive in 97% of cases [4].

Clinical Examination

Examination of the hip must assess the functional status of the hip, the range of movement, the response to specific provocative manoeuvres and sources of extra-articular pain.

Examination of the hip should begin with the patient walking assessing the gait and in particular the stride length, duration of stance phase and coronal and sagittal balance. The patient should next stand and inspection is performed from in front, the side and behind for scars, asymmetry and deformity before performing the Trendelenburg's test. Next the patient is made to lie supine on the examining couch and true leg length is assessed measuring from the anterior superior iliac spine to the medial malleolus. Palpation begins with palpation of the groin starting at the pubic symphysis before proceeding to the midpoint of the inguinal ligament to palpate for a hernial cough impulse, the iliopsoas tendon, the adductor tendon, and then to the greater trochanter, the anterior superior iliac spine and the ischial tuberosity for tenderness. At this point it is simple to perform the Thomas's test for fixed flexion deformity before continuing to examine active and passive hip movements. Flexion must be assessed and then on returning to 90° flexion, external and internal rotation can be measured which is then repeated in the neutral position. Abduction and adduction must be measured with a hand on the iliac crest to palpate for pelvic tilt disguising a true limitation of hip movement. The impingement test can be performed next flexing, adduction and internally rotating the hip bringing the anterior femoral neck into contact with the anterosuperior acetabulum provoking pain in the presence of a anterior labral or chondral pathology.

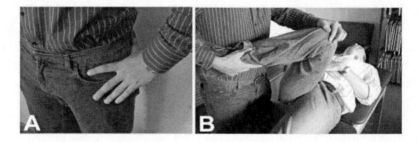

Figure 1. Positive C-sign: The patients indicates the location of pain by gripping the lateral hip with the thumb on the posterior aspect of the greater trochanter and the fingers resting on the groin (A). The impingement test is performed by adducting and internally rotating the hip in 90 degrees of flexion, bringing the anterior femoral neck into contact with the anterosuperior acetabulum provoking pain in the presence of an anterior labral or chondral pathology (B).

(Figure 1-B) The FABER (Flexion Abduction External Rotation) test provokes pain when the hip is rotated in the abducted position, opposing the anterior superior rim of the femoral neck to the superior acetabulum and is also a useful special test to perform before making a final assessment of the neurovascular status of the limb.

We suggest that the above physical examination is performed in a routine and a systematic manner and that a positive impingement test is highly suggestive of intra-articular hip pathology.

Investigations

The main imaging modalities used to assess the painful hip are plain radiographs, computed tomography (CT) and magnetic resonance imaging with (MRA) and without intra-articular contrast (non-contrast MRI). In addition to imaging a diagnostic hip injection of local anaesthetic can be used to confirm that pain is indeed intra-articular in origin.

Plain radiograph is routinely employed to assess patients for evidence of osteoarthritis, the presence of the crossover sign and the ischial spine sign indicative of acetabular retroversion suggesting pincer type of impingement. The cross-table lateral view is examined for the presence of an asphericity of the femoral head suggesting a cam impingement lesion on the anterior femoral neck and the alpha angle can be measured for quantification.

MRI is routinely used to assess the painful hip for labral and chondral injury particularly where hip arthroscopy is being considered. While the sensitivity and specificity of MRI techniques reported varies widely depending on study design, experience of the radiologists and MRI sequencing used we find the negative predictive value of MRI to rule out intra-articular pathology when the MRI is normal of particular use. While a number of studies are strongly supportive of MRA, a review of 92 patients having non-contrast MRI of the hip and hip arthroscopy, musculoskeletal radiologists identified over 94% of labral tears subsequently diagnosed at surgery with 92% inter-observer agreement and similar results reported for chondral lesions [5]. The authors suggest that these results with non-contrast MRI were achieved due to a small pixel size and a fast spin sequence. Certainly imaging of the chondral surface with current MR sequencing remains less sensitive than the assessment of the acetabular labrum. Also, an earlier paper comparing MRI findings with hip arthroscopic findings in 23 patients investigated for undiagnosed hip pain proved the MRI accurate for diagnosing labral tears and the presence of loose bodies but less reliable for assessment of chondral surfaces for softening and degeneration [6].

Beaule et al recommended routine use of three-dimensional computed tomography to assess the bony anatomy of the femoral head-neck junction prior to hip arthroscopy [7]. In our experience the presence of the impingement lesion can be reliably detected on a crosstable lateral radiograph of the hip and the MR radial sequences and subsequently confirmed at arthroscopy at which point osteoplasty can be performed without exposing the patient to a huge amount of radiation and prolonged costly imaging techniques.

Where diagnostic uncertainty remains following appropriate imaging we have a low threshold to use a fluoroscopically guided diagnostic hip injection of local anaesthetic to confirm that the hip joint is the source of the patients pain.

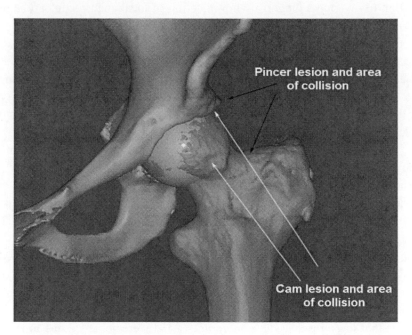

Figure 2. 3D-reconstructed view demonstrating location and area of collision in cam- and pincer-type femoroacetebular impingement.

Byrd and Jones reported a 90% positive predictive value of diagnostic hip injection in a series of 40 hip arthroscopies 8 however complete relief of pain is not always achieved and the response does correlate to the severity of pathology and presence of other contiguous extra-articular problems as demonstrated by Martin et al reporting that 37% of patients with a proven labral tear had a <50% improvement in hip symptoms following intra-articular injection [9,10].

We recommend that the routine use of AP pelvis and cross table lateral radiograph in addition to simple non-contrast MRI interpreted by a musculoskeletal radiologist for all patients with hip pain where hip arthroscopy is being considered. Where diagnostic uncertainty persists a diagnostic injection of local anaesthetic using fluoroscopic guidance is recommended before proceeding to arthroscopy.

TECHNIQUE

Hip arthroscopy can be successfully performed using the supine and the lateral position. However, for the purpose of this chapter, we will describe the technique in the supine position. The supine position allows for distraction of the hip joint by using a standard installation on a classical fracture table. An oversized (12-16 cm outer diameter) perineal post is applied at the operative side. The perineal post is positioned in proximity of the groin, but without direct contact to avoid iatrogenic damage to the pudendal nerve [11]. The contralateral extremity is abducted as necessary to allow for unobstructed use of the image intensifier during the procedure. (Figure 3) When the image intensifier is rotated 30-45°, a clear view of the anterolateral femur can be obtained, showing the anatomical location of anomalies of the proximal femur.

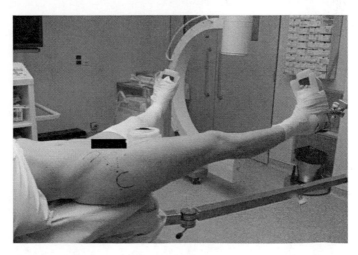

Figure 3. Patient installation in supine position on a classical fracture table. An oversized perineal post is applied at the operative side. The contralateral extremity is abducted as necessary to allow unobstructed use of the image intensifier.

Access to the Central and Peripheral Compartments of the Hip

The operative hip is positioned in neutral abduction-adduction. Increased adduction during prolonged procedures can cause pressure sores at the side of the perineal post [12]. The leg is then held in slight flexion and neutral rotation to relax the anterior capsule to facilitate access to the peripheral compartment. Finally, the traction table is tilted in slight Trendelenburg to use the patient body as a counterforce during distraction. The positioning of the leg on the leg holder should allow for further flexing of the leg further during the assessment of the peripheral compartment.

Proper positioning of the patient is then controlled by applying traction under fluoroscopic guidance prior to commencement of the procedure. We aim for a distraction of at least 1cm for safe intra-articular access. A vacuum phenomenon, visible on fluoroscopy, will appear with the application of increasing traction. If adequate distraction is not readily achieved, some time should be allowed for stress relaxation of the elastic tissues holding the joint in place to occur and over distraction should be avoided. In case of over distraction, a sudden and usually extensive displacement of the femur head can occur. When adequate distraction of the hip joint has been obtained, anatomical landmarks necessary for portal placement are marked on the skin before traction is released. The hip is then prepped and draped, and distraction is reapplied at the start of the procedure.

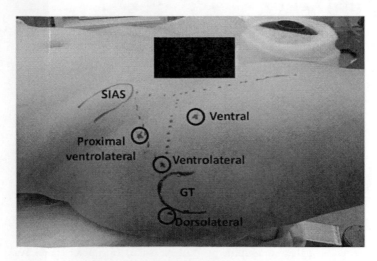

Figure 4. Commonly used portals in the supine approach to the central and peripheral compartment of the hip.

Access to the joint is achieved by pre-positioning of an 18-gauge needle under fluoroscopic guidance. The needle is aimed at the acetabular fossa, which can only be achieved by passing close to the superior tip of the greater trochanter.

The anterolateral portal is usually placed first and, unlike the following portals, without direct arthroscopic control. It is therefore advisable to use blunt tools, to avoid damage to the joint cartilage and to enter the joint at an adequate distance from the acetabular rim to avoid penetration of the acetabular labrum. An overview of the most commonly used portals is provided in Figure 4.

If the psoas tendon needs to be assessed, care should be taken not to internally rotate the leg as this moves the tendon and its insertion to the lesser trochanter, medially and posteriorly, impeding access to this structure.

Access to the Lateral Compartment

To access the surgical compartment between the fascia lata and the greater trochanter, the leg is placed in 30-40° of abduction. No traction is required. The abduction of the leg relaxes the iliotibial band, fascia lata and tensor fascia and gluteus maximus muscles. In addition, pressured flow during the arthroscopic procedure will aid in maintaining an unobstructed view of this compartment. Figure 5 demonstrates patient positioning and commonly used portals to access the lateral compartment.

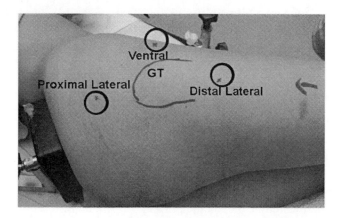

Figure 5. Commonly used portals in the supine approach to the lateral compartment of the hip.

INDICATIONS

Operative arthroscopy about the hip is becoming an increasingly well-recognized procedure. With increased implementation of the procedure, advancements in endoscopic instrumentation and techniques, the pathology that can now be addressed arthroscopically has grown significantly [51].

The most common indication by far is femoroacetabular impingement (FAI) of the hip. FAI is defined as non-physiological abutment of the femoral neck against the acetabular rim causing damage to the acetabular labrum and articular cartilage. FAI has become a well-recognized pathogenic factor in the natural course of idiopathic hip osteoarthritis, and arthroscopic treatment might delay or prevent the extent of such evolution [13]. The condition usually occurs in the presence of a structural anomaly at the femur head-neck junction (cam impingement) and/or acetabular rim (pincer impingement). Depending on the source, the prevalence of these anatomical malformations ranges from 4.3% to 48% in men and from 3.6 to 31% in women [14, 15]. Arthroscopic treatment involves repair or debridement of the resultant intra-articular lesions with concomitant correction of the anomalous bony anatomy. (Figure 6)

Intra-articular access, as commonly used for FAI, can also easily serve as a minimally invasive alternative to address other, usually less prevalent conditions, including loose body removal (synovial chondromatosis), ligamentum teres tears (partial or complete) and lavage and debridement in case of early osteoarthritis or septic arthritis.

Intracapsular arthroscopic access to the femur neck area, without distracting the joint can also be useful for synovial biopsy in inflammatory arthritis where a diagnosis cannot be confirmed and for the diagnostic work-up of a total hip replacement or painful hip resurfacing [49] where ALVAL and excessive metal wear cannot be demonstrated [16, 17].

A frequently performed procedure, both open and arthroscopic, involves release of the psoas tendon. This is indicated for therapy-resistant painful internal snapping or for impingement of the tendon in case of an anteverted acetabular component in hip arthroplasty. (Figure 7) The release can be performed either endoscopically at the level of the iliopsoas tendon insertion at the lesser trochanter, or at the level of the hip joint, by approaching the tendon through the joint capsule. Both techniques have been shown to provide an equal and beneficial clinical outcome [18,19]. Again, no distraction is required to perform these releases.

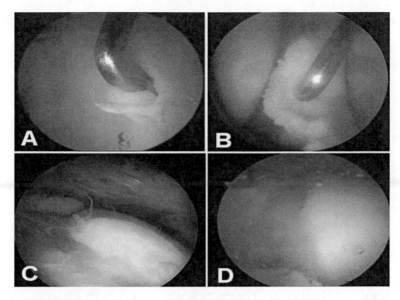

Figure 6. Intra-articular findings in case of FAI can range from small (A) to extensive (B) chondral lesions. Cam lesions at the femoral head-neck junction (C) need to be identified and surgically corrected to restore offset (D) and to avoid ongoing impingement.

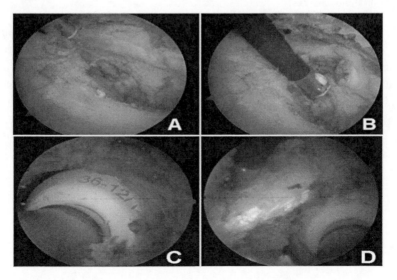

Figure 7. Release of the psoas tendon can be indicated for therapy-resistent painful internal snapping (A-B) or for impingement of the tendon in case of an anteverted acetabular component in hip arthroplasty (C-D).

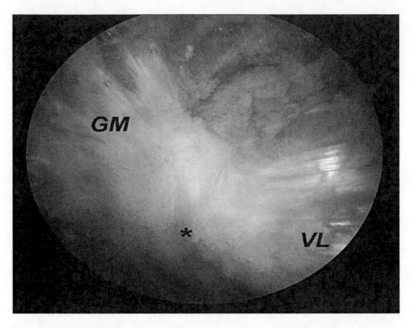

Figure 8. Endoscopic approach to the lateral compartment of the hip. Image shows view on the greater trochanter (asterisk) and insertion of the vastus lateralis (VL) and medial glutal muscle (GM).

Finally, more and more attention is being paid to the peri trochanteric space or the lateral compartment. This compartment can be approached for release of the iliotibial band (ITB), restoration 'rotator cuff' of the hip i.e. painful gluteal tears at the side of the greater trochanter and in cases of recalcitrant greater trochanteric pain syndrome [20]. (Figure 8) As the peri-trochanteric space lies adjacent to the piriformis tendon and sciatic nerve in the deep gluteal region, recent reports have shown that the established arthroscopic portals for access to the lateral compartment also allow for endoscopic assessment and, if necessary, release of the sciatic nerve in the cases of entrapment [21].

COMPLICATIONS AND CONTRAINDICATIONS

As mentioned previously, hip arthroscopy has evolved significantly in recent years in terms of equipment, surgical technique and operative skill resulting in a reduction in complication rates. However, complications do occur from time to time and can be broadly divided into those related to traction, irrigation and trauma.

In a review of 73 patients undergoing hip arthroscopy for severe hip pain with an average traction time of 58 minutes (30 – 150 minutes range) 16.4% had trauma to the femoral head by the arthroscope [22]. To reduce the incidence of this traumatic complication it is recommended to distract the hip joint by 1cm with traction and to guide the cannula into the hip using fluoroscopic guidance and gentle rotational movements (23=ref for 1cm distraction).

In a large retrospective review of 530 hip arthroscopies 20 transient neuropraxias relating to positioning and prolonged distraction times were reported, with a 7% transient sciatic neuropraxia rate in a smaller study and <1% neuropraxia rate in a large series of 640 consecutive hip arthroscopies [22, 24]. These series with high rates of neuropraxia are related to prolonged and excessive traction but these resolved spontaneously in all cases [22,23,25]. The low rate in the latter study is attributed to 'trial of traction' with initial distraction after lateral positioning with fluoroscopic guidance to visualise the degree of subluxation before traction is released while the patient is prepared and draped and reapplied for central compartment arthroscopy. It is also important in the lateral position to avoid excessive lateral force due to the risk of perineal tears that have been reported in a large series [26].

Extravasation of irrigation fluid is another important complication that must be anticipated and recognised with increased risk associated with prolonged and extra-articular surgery and where high irrigation pressures are applied [22, 27]. In a single case of cardiac arrest following arthroscopy to remove a loose body in a patient with recent acetabular fracture a clear pathway is present from the hip allowing irrigation fluid to be absorbed systemically but extravasation can occur by less obvious paths [28]. During an arthroscopy on a 15-year-old patient lasting 105 minutes the patient became hypothermic intra-operatively and post-operatively developed abdominal pain and neurological disturbance with 2500ml of irrigation fluid visualised on abdominal ultrasound [29]. It was hypothesised that the fluid may have tracked along the iliopsoas muscle and iliac vessels before perforating the peritoneum in this case where the symptoms settled without treatment the next day. One episode of irrigation fluid extravasation was reported in a small series of 19 hip arthroscopies where surgery was performed under regional anaesthesia and was terminated after the patient reported significant abdominal pain [27].

Other complications reported in large series include port site bleeding, port site haematoma, instrument breakage and trochanteric bursitis with an overall 1.6% risk including all complications [26]. Another large study reported an overall 1.4% overall complication rate in 1054 patients but this did exclude the 30 hips (2.8%) that could not be accessed due to severe dysplasia or osteoarthritis potentially increasing the complication rate to 4.2% when these are included [30].

The risk of complications from hip arthroscopy can be minimised by careful positioning with padding of supports and a 'trial of traction' to reduce the traction time and the risk of neurological sequelae. Instrumentation should be used judiciously and with care under fluoroscopic guidance to an adequately distracted hip joint and pressure should be minimised to reduce the risk of fluid extravasation.

The absolute contraindications are hip ankylosis, superficial or deep infection and overlying wounds or ulcers with relative contraindications including gross obesity, severe hip joint destruction and recent fracture [30].

OUTCOMES

Hip arthroscopy is a relatively new branch of orthopaedic surgery that is rapidly gaining popularity as results are published supporting its use. While at the outset it primarily addressed pathology in athletes its use is now increasingly generic successfully treating common conditions affecting the general population.

The follow-up of results for hip arthroscopy remains limited to 10 years follow-up and study groups remain small. Generally studies concern individual patient groups and various modes of treatment including debridement versus repair or labrum tears and debridement versus osteoplasty for cam impingement lesions. Fundamental to outcome in all these studies is patient selection. Numerous studies demonstrate that any early clinical or radiological evidence of osteoarthritis or chondral tears significantly reduces potential improvement in patient symptoms and outcome assessed with various outcome scores including the modified Harris Hip Score [32-37]. A retrospective review of 56 arthroscopies of the central compartment of the hip showed that outcome and patient satisfaction were primarily determined by grade of cartilage damage [38].

Patients with a hip joint space <2mm have also been shown to be 39 times more likely to progress to early hip arthroplasty [35, 39]. Patient satisfaction remains acceptable with studies suggesting that 80% of patients would undergo the same procedure again and 68% improved at 72 months with no complaint in daily or sporting activities [40].

Several studies address some individual patient groups of particular interest. Athletes have had excellent results from hip arthroscopy in terms of return to professional sport. In a series of 6 professional football players, 5 returned to professional sport at a mean of 12 months following anterior labrum debridement for unstable traumatic labrum tears [41]. Philippon reported on the return to sport of 45 professional athletes who underwent arthroscopic treatment for FAI with 93% returning to the professional level [34]. In a study of predominantly female adolescent patients with a mean age of 15, all having labral pathology, 5 with pincer impingement, 2 with isolated cam and 9 with mixed pathology of which 7 underwent suture anchor repair and 9 patients underwent partial labral debridement 39=10. Mean patient satisfaction score was 9 with significant improvement in modified Harris Hip Score following surgery [42].

Longer-term follow-up data is now available for patients with labrum tears. A 10-year follow-up study with 100% follow-up of 50 patients who had a hip arthroscopy for labral tears 10 year ago has recently reported their outcomes [37]. For patients without arthritis at the time of the index procedure the median improvement in the modified Harris Hip Score was 35 with 85% continuing to show a significant improvement at 10 years. Another smaller 10 year follow-up study with 10 patients demonstrated a median improvement on the modified Harris Hip Score of 25 points with the maximal benefit noticed in first month and plateauing in month [32].

Osteoplasty for symptomatic cam impingement is a recent advance in hip arthroscopy and is superior to arthroscopic debridement and no surgical intervention although both treatments have been shown to improve patients overall in terms of function and pain sub-scores [43]. A prospective study of 122 patients with femoroacetabular impingement and positive impingement tests demonstrated patient satisfaction scores of 9/10 where 47 patients underwent a microfracture of femoral head, 30 of the acetabular surface and 9 for both and good to excellent outcome in 75% of hips at a minimum of 1 year follow-up [33].

Several systematic reviews have been performed recently demonstrating satisfactory overall outcomes following hip arthroscopy. In a systematic review of literature between January 1980 and September 2005, Robertson reviewed articles that concerned patient satisfaction following arthroscopic acetabular labral debridement [44]. In conclusion, over two thirds of patients were satisfied with the outcome of acetabular labral debridement at a mean follow-up of 3.5 years and a complete resolution of mechanical symptoms in those patients with this complaint [44]. This relatively low rate of satisfaction is criticised by some suggesting that labral repair should be attempted where possible as suggested by results in Espinosa's study with superior clinical and radiological outcome in patients with labral repair versus labral debridement [45]. Another systematic review including 19 relevant articles where patients were managed with open and arthroscopic surgery for labral tears and femoroacetabular impingement demonstrated a range of 67-93% good to excellent outcomes in the arthroscopic group [46]. In a recent systematic review of FAI an improvement in function of 68-96% over a short-term follow-up (mean 3.2 years) was noted. Conversion to total hip arthroplasty in this study was reported in 0% to 26% of the cases [39].

Further studies are required to clarify the patient sub-group that benefits most from hip arthroscopy and to determine the best treatment for individual indications. Patients with a symptomatic traumatic labral tear in the absence of chondral damage or associated osteoarthritis are likely to improve with arthroscopic surgery though it is less clear which tears should be repaired versus those that should be debrided. Results of osteoplasty for femoroacetabular impingement are encouraging although it must be realised that this patient group is likely to have associated labral tears and chondral damage and are therefore at a relatively high risk of developing osteoarthritis and may require early hip arthroplasty despite arthroscopy. While patient selection is paramount, hip arthroscopy improves pain and function for a young active group of patients with a variety of underlying intra and extra-articular pathology.

FUTURE PERSPECTIVES

Femoroacetabular impingement (FAI) is by far the most common arthroscopically addressed condition by the hip arthroscopist and has recently been identified as a precursor to osteoarthritis of the hip [50]. Both morphological abnormality and functional overuse of the hip joint have been associated with the progression to osteoarthritis, but clear case identification remains challenging. According to recent literature, up to 74% of healthy persons demonstrate radiological signs related to FAI [14]. These numbers make apparent that the diagnosis of this complex disorder is more multifaceted than simple evaluation of femoral head sphericity or acetabular coverage.

Furthermore, concerns have been raised about the accuracy and timing of surgical treatment and the related prognosis, thus highlighting the importance of improving not only the diagnostics and treatment, but also the understanding of the underlying pathological condition. Improved diagnosis and patient selection, in combination with increased surgical accuracy, are therefore the main challenges facing the hip arthroscopist today.

Both industry and academic researchers have started to focus on simulation platforms, computer-aided systems, including robotics and navigational systems and virtual surgical planning and training tools to improve the diagnosis and to increase the rate of successful operations [47,48]. Different techniques allowing for virtual planning have now been development. They involve assessment of hip morphology, hip range of motion or a combination of both. The virtual plan can then be translated into the operating room using standard navigational assistance. (Figure 9) In addition, the first studies have become available demonstrating that surgical accuracy in performing the surgical plan can even be augmented by robotic assistance. Technology in assisting hip arthroscopy is rapidly advancing. However, it remains to be established whether it will improve early clinical results and long term prognosis of patients in relation to the development of osteoarthritis.

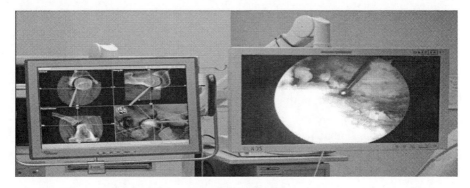

Figure 9. Virtual planning and computer–aided hip arthroscopy for femoroacetabular impingement.

Research is also being directly towards finding solutions to articular cartilage lesions in the hip and addressing these lesions arthroscopically. Reconstruction of the ligamentum teres, bone grafting of acetabular and femoral cysts, grafting of the acetabular labrum with the tensor fascia lata graft, arthroscopic-assisted partial resurfacings of the hip, arthroscopic release of rectus femoris and arthroscopic release of the sciatic nerve are some of the novel techniques that are being attempted and performed in small numbers in centers around the world. However, it is certainly not difficult to envisage that these techniques will be well established and be performed routinely in the not too distant future.

In conclusion, the future of arthroscopic hip surgery is bright and there is no doubt that we have come a long way from 1931 when Burman stated that 'it was manifestly impossible to insert a needle between the head of the femur and the acetabulum'. However, it is a procedure not without complications and has a steep learning curve and therefore appropriate training is essential prior to embarking on the same [51].

REFERENCES

[1]   O'Leary J, Berend K, Vail T. The relationship between diagnosis and outcome in arthroscopy of the hip. *Arthroscopy*. 2001;17-181-188.

[2]   Byrd J. Hip Arthroscopy: Patient Assessment and Indications. *AAOS Instructional Course Lectures*. 2003;52:711-719.

[3]   Burnett R et al. Clinical presentation of patients with tears of the acetabular labrum. *JBJS(Am)*. 2006;88A(7):1448-1457.

[4]   Philipon M. *Clinical presentation of femoroacetbular impingement*. Knee Surgical Sports Traumatology Association. 2007;15:1041-1047.

[5]   Mintz D et al. Magnetic resonance imaging of the hip: detection of labral and chondral abnormalities using noncontrast imaging. Arthroscopy: *The Journal of Arthroscopic and Related Surgery*. 2005;21(4):385-393.

[6]   Edwards D, Lomas D, Villar R. Diagnosis of the painful hip by magnetic resonance imaging and arthroscopy. *JBJS*. 1995;77B:374-376.

[7]   Beaule P et al. Three-dimensional computed tomography of the hip in the assessment of femoroacetabular impingement. *Journal of Orthopaedic Research*. 2005;23:1286-1292.

[8] Byrd J. Diagnostic accuracy of clinical assessment, magnetic resonance arthrography and intra-articular injection in hip arthroscopy patients. *American Journal of Sports Medicine*. 2004;32:1668.

[9] 1(2): Byrd J, Jones K. Prospective analysis of hip arthroscopy with a 2 year follow-up. *Arthroscopy*. 2000;16:578-587.

[10] Martin R. The diagnostic accuracy of a clinical examination in determining intra-articular hip pain for potential arthroscopy candidates. Arthroscopy: *The Journal of Arthroscopic and Related Surgery*. 2008;24(9):1013-1018.

[11] Hip arthroscopy utilizing the supine position. Byrd JW. *Arthroscopy*. 1994 Jun;10(3):275-80.

[12] Diagnostic and operative arthroscopy of the hip.Eriksson E, Arvidsson I, Arvidsson H. *Orthopedics*. 1986 Feb;9(2):169-76.

[13] The etiology of osteoarthritis of the hip: an integrated mechanical concept. Ganz R, Leunig M, Leunig-Ganz K, Harris WH. *Clin. Orthop. Relat. Res*. 2008 Feb;466(2):264-72.

[14] Computed tomography assessment of hip joints in asymptomatic individuals in relation to femoroacetabular impingement. Kang AC, Gooding AJ, Coates MH, Goh TD, Armour P, Rietveld J. *Am. J. Sports Med*. 2010 Jun;38(6):1160-5.

[15] The prevalence of cam-type deformity of the hip joint: a survey of 4151 subjects of the Copenhagen Osteoarthritis Study. Gosvig KK, Jacobsen S, Sonne-Holm S, Gebuhr P. *Acta Radiol*. 2008 May;49(4):436-41.

[16] Hip arthroscopy in patients with painful hip following resurfacing arthroplasty. Pattyn C, Verdonk R, Audenaert E. *Knee Surg Sports Traumatol Arthrosc*. 2011 Mar 16. [Epub ahead of print].

[17] Diagnostic arthroscopy of the hip joint in pigmented villonodular synovitis. Janssens X, Van Meirhaeghe J, Verdonk R, Verjans P, Cuvelier C, Veys EM. *Arthroscopy*. 1987;3(4):283-7.

[18] Arthroscopic psoas tenotomy. Wettstein M, Jung J, Dienst M. *Arthroscopy*. 2006 Aug;22(8):907.e1-4.

[19] Prospective randomized study of 2 different techniques for endoscopic iliopsoas tendon release in the treatment of internal snapping hip syndrome. Ilizaliturri VM Jr, Chaidez C, Villegas P, Briseño A, Camacho-Galindo J. *Arthroscopy*. 2009 Feb;25(2):159-63.

[20] Endoscopic repair of gluteus medius tendon tears of the hip. Voos JE, Shindle MK, Pruett A, Asnis PD, Kelly BT. *Am. J. Sports Med*. 2009 Apr;37(4):743-7.

[21] The endoscopic treatment of sciatic nerve entrapment/deep gluteal syndrome. Martin HD, Shears SA, Johnson JC, Smathers AM, Palmer IJ. *Arthroscopy.* 2011 Feb;27(2):172-81.

[22] Lo Y. Complications of hip arthroscopy: analysis of seventy three cases. *Chang Gung Medical Journal.* 2006;29(1):86-91.

[23] McCarthy J, Lee J. Hip Arthroscopy. Indications and Technical Pearls. *Clinical Orthopaedics and Related Research.* 2005;441:180-187.

[24] Sampson T. Compications of hip arthroscopy. *Clinics in Sports Medicine.* 2001;20(4):831-835.

[25] Brumback R et al. Pudendal nerve palsy complicating intramedullary nailing of the femur. *JBJS(Am).* 1992;74:1450-5.

[26] Griffin D, Villar R. Complications of arthroscopy of the hip. *JBJS(Br).* 1999;81:604-606.

[27] Funke E, Munzinger U. Complications in hip arthroscopy. Arthroscopy: *The Journal of Arthroscopic and Related Surgery.* 1996;12(2):156-159.

[28] Bartlett C et al. Cardiac arrest as a result of intraabdominal extravasation of fluid during arthroscopic removal of a loose body from the hip joint of a patient with an acetabular fracture. *Journal of Orthopaedic Trauma.* 1998;12:294-299.

[29] Haupt U et al. Intra- and retroperitoneal irrigation liquid after arthroscopy of the hip. Arthroscopy: *The Journal of Arthroscopic and Related Surgery.* 2008;24(8):966-968.

[30] Clarke M, Arora A, Villar R. Hip arthroscopy: Complications in 1054 cases. *Clinical Orthopaedics and Related Research.* 2003;406:84-88.

[31] Bharam S. Clincal evaluation of hip pain: indications and coniraindications. *Operative Techniques in Orthopaedics.* 2005;175.

[32] 32. Byrd J, Jones K. Prospective analysis of hip arthroscopy with 10 year follow-up. *Clinical Orthopaedics and Related Research.* 2010;468: 741-746.

[33] Larson C, Giveans M. Arthroscopic management of femoroacetabular impingement: Early outcome measure. Arthroscopy: *The Journal of Arthroscopic and Related Research.* 2008;24(5):540-546.

[34] Philippon M et al. *Outcomes following hip arthroscopy for femoroacetabular impingement with associated chondrolabral dysfunction.* 2009;91-B(1): 16-23.

[35] Phillippon M et al. Arthroscopy for femoroacetabular impingement in the athlete. *Clinics in sports medicine*. 2006. 25(2): 399-308.

[36] Clohisy J et al. Surgical treatment of femoroacetabular impingement. *Clinical Orthopaedic and Related Research*. 2010. 468:555-564.

[37] Byrd J, Jones K. Hip arthroscopy for labral pathology: prospective analysis with 10 year follow-up. Arthroscopy: *The Journal of Arthroscopic and Related Surgery*. 2009. 25(4): 365-368.

[38] Londers J, Van Melkebeek J. Hip Arthroscopy: Outcome and patient satisfaction after 5-10 years. *Acta Orthop. Belg*. 2007;73:478-483.

[39] Chan Y et al. Evaluating hip labral tears using magnetic resonance arthrography: a prospective study comparing hip arthroscopy and magnetic resonance arthrography diagnosis. Arthroscopy: *The Journal of Arthroscopic and Related Surgery*. 2005;21(10):1250e1-1250e10.

[40] O'Leary J et al. The diagnosis between diagnosis and outcome in arthroscopy of the hip. Arthroscopy: *The Journal of Arthroscopic and Related Surgery*. 2001. 17(2): 181-188.

[41] Saw T, Villar R. Footballer's hip: A report of six cases. *JBJS(Br)*. 2004;86:655-658.

[42] Philippon et al. Early outcomes after hip arthroscopy for femoroacetabular impingement in the athletic adolescant patient: a preliminary report. *Journal of Pediatric Orthopaedics*. 2008. 28(7):705-710.

[43] Bardakos N et al. Early outcome of hip arthroscopy for femoroacetabular impingement. The role of femoral osteoplasty in symptomatic improvement. *JBJS*. 2008. 90-B:1570-5.

[44] Robertson W et al. Arthroscopic management of labral tears in the hip. A systematic review. *Clinical Orthopaedics and Related Research*. 2006;455:88-92.

[45] Espinosa N et al. Treatment of femoroacetabular impingement: preliminary results of labral refixation: surgical technique. *JBJS(Am)*. 2006;88A:925-35.

[46] Bedi A et al. Systematic Review. The management of labral tears and femoroacetabular impingement of the hip in the young, active patient. Arthroscopy: *The Journal of Orthopaedic and Related Surgery*. 2008;24(10): 1135-1145.

[47] A method for three-dimensional evaluation and computer aided treatment of femoroacetabular impingement. Audenaert E, Vigneron L, Pattyn C. *Comput. Aided Surg.* 2011;16(3):143-8.

[48] Kather J, Hagen ME, Morel P, Fasel J, Markar S, Schueler M.Robotic hip arthroscopy in human anatomy. *Int. J. Med. Robot.* 2010 Sep;6(3):301-5.

[49] The role of arthroscopy in resurfacing arthroplasty of the hip. Khanduja V, Villar RN. *Arthroscopy.* 2008 Jan;24(1):122.e1-3. Epub 2007 Apr 19.

[50] The arthroscopic management of femoroacetabular impingement. Khanduja V, Villar RN. *Knee Surg. Sports Traumatol. Arthrosc.* 2007 Aug;15(8):1035-40. Epub 2007 May 30.

[51] Arthroscopic surgery of the hip: current concepts and recent advances. Khanduja V, Villar RN. *J. Bone Joint Surg. Br.* 2006 Dec;88(12):1557-66.

In: Arthroscopy
Editors: K. Elani et al.

ISBN: 978-1-61470-955-8
© 2012 Nova Science Publishers, Inc.

Chapter IV

Wrist Arthroscopy: Arthroscopic Repair of Avulsed Triangular Fibrocartilage Complex to the Fovea of the Distal Ulna-

Norimasa Iwasaki[*]

Department of Orthopedic Surgery, Hokkaido University
School of Medicine, Japan

ABSTRACT

The triangular fibrocartilage complex (TFCC) plays an important role in stabilizing the distal radioulnar joint (DRUJ) during forearm rotation. Therefore, tears of the TFCC lead to varying degrees of DRUJ instability and to symptomatic conditions of the wrist. The ulnar end of the TFCC consists of 3 components, including the proximal triangular ligament, the distal hammock structure, and the ulnar collateral ligament. Among the 3 components, the proximal triangular ligament represents the

[*] Department of Orthopedic Surgery, Hokkaido University School of Medicine, Kita 15, Nishi 7, Sapporo 060-8638, Japan. Phone: 81-11-706-5937, Fax: 81-11-706-6054, Email: niwasaki@med.hokudai.ac.jp.

deep component (dc-TFCC) inserting into the fovea adjacent to the articular surface of the distal ulna (ulnar fovea). Recent anatomical and biomechanical studies have demonstrated that the TFCC insertion into the fovea of the distal ulna has a greater effect on DRUJ stability than other insertion sites. Therefore, surgical reattachment against avulsion of the foveal TFCC insertion must be considered to achieve stability for the DRUJ. Although open techniques of reattachment for avulsed dc-TFCC to the ulna have been introduced, arthroscopic repair techniques have not been established because of technical difficulties. To address this concern, we developed a new technique of arthroscopic reattachment of the avulsed dc-TFCC into the ulnar fovea. In this chapter, we mainly introduce previous open and our arthroscopic procedures for the treatment of this lesion.

INTRODUCTION

In 1920, Prof. Kenji Takagi [1] first reported large joint arthroscopy. Then, Prof. Takagi successfully developed arthroscopic systems for smaller joint surgeries. In 1985, Whipple and Powell [2] performed a series of cadaveric studies to establish a coordinated system of portals for arthroscopic access to the radiocarpal joint, the midcarpal joint, and the distal radioulnar joint (DRUJ) . Based on these studies, Whipple undertook successful clinical trials of wrist arthroscopy. Since the initial clinical trials, wrist arthroscopy has developed into an essential diagnostic and therapeutic tool. Currently, wrist arthroscopy is recommended for a wide range of wrist disorders, which had been treated with open procedures (Table 1). Wrist arthroscopy, especially, has become the gold standard in the diagnosis and treatment of triangular fibrocartilage complex (TFCC) lesions. As space is limited, this chapter focuses on arthroscopic surgical procedures for the treatment of the deep component of TFCC, which plays a critical role in the stability of the DRUJ.

TYPES OF WRIST ARTHROSCOPY

Generally, wrist arthroscopy includes radiocarpal joint, midcarpal joint, and DRUJ. The techniques used in radiocarpal joint and DRUJ arthroscopy are mentioned later. Although pathology examined by midcarpal joint arthroscopy is less than that by radiocarpal joint arthroscopy, much diagnostic information can be obtained from arthroscopic examination of this interval.

Table 1. Indications for Wrist Arthroscopic Surgery

Procedure	Target Tissue or Disease	
Resection or Debridment	Dorsal/volar ganglion	Carpal bones
	Interosseous ligaments	Distal ulna/ulnar styloid
	TFCC tear	Radial styloid
	Synovitis	Free bodies
	Cartilaginous lesions	
Release	Volar/dorsal capsular release	
Shrinkage	Thermal shrinkage of capsule/ligament shrinkage	
Repair	Radiocarpal ligament	Distal radius fracture
	Scapholunate instability	Perilunate dislocation
	Lunotriquetral instability	Scaphoid fracture
	TFCC repair	
Reconstruction	Scapholunate ligament reconstruction	Partial wrist fusions
	DRUJ stabilization	Scaphoid nonunion bone graft

The arthroscope is usually introduced into the midcarpal space between the scaphoid and capitate (radial midcarpal portal). The articular surface of the scaphocapitate joint to the scaphotrapeziotrapezoid (STT) joint is observed. Osteoarthritic changes are often observed in the STT articular surface. The severity may be assessed by probing the articular surface with a probe through the STT portal. The scapholunate interval is also observed. Degenerative changes in the articular cartilage along the margins of the scaphoid and lunate indicate the existence of scaphoid rotatory subluxation. This is a significant finding for the diagnosis of scapholunate dissociation. The lunotriquetral interval is also examined for symmetry. The gap of this interval is normally the same width volar to dorsal. The articulation between the hamate and the triquetrum is held very tight by the volar triquetro-hamate-capitate ligament. The widening of this interval by traction or radial deviation indicates midcarpal instability. An articular defect on the extreme proximal pole of the hamate is another finding of midcarpal instability. The ulnar capsule of the midcarpal joint should be examined for detecting synovitis. A probe or other instrument is introduced at the articular junction of the lunate, triquetrum, hamate, and capitate (ulnar midcarpal portal), if probing or shaving is required in this region.

ANATOMY OF THE **TFCC**

The TFCC interposes between the proximal carpal row and the distal end of the ulna. It had been thought to consist of fibrocartilage, ligament, and joint capsule connecting the distal radius, distal ulna, and the ulnar aspect of the carpal bones that separates the DRUJ from the radiocarpal joint under normal circumstances. However, histological and anatomical research has demonstrated that the TFCC has complex anatomical characteristics contributing to the stability of the DRUJ [3,4].

The ulnar side of the TFCC is composed of 3 components, including the proximal triangular ligament, the distal hammock structure, and the ulnar collateral ligament [5-7]. Among them, the distal hammock structure and the ulnar collateral ligament are considered as the superficial component of the TFCC (sc-TFCC) inserting directly into the ulnar styloid. On the other hand, the proximal triangular ligament represents the deep component of the TFCC (dc-TFCC) inserting into the fovea of the distal ulna (ulnar fovea) (Figure 1) [5,6,8]. The longitudinal axis of forearm rotation passes through the center of the radial head proximally and through the ulnar fovea distally. The fovea is the recess lying between the hyaline cartilage of the ulna pole and the ulna styloid. The proximal triangular ligament spans to the volar- and dorsal-ulnar corners of the distal radius with 2 limbs.

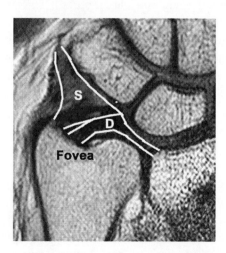

Figure 1. Coronal MRI view of the ulnar wrist. S, superficial component of the TFCC (sc-TFCC) inserting directly into the ulnar styloid. D, deep component of the TFCC (dc-TFCC) inserting into the fovea of the distal ulna.

STABILITY OF THE DRUJ BY TFCC

The radius of curvature of the sigmoid notch is greater than that of the seat of the ulna. This bony incongruity of artcular surfaces lead to a geometrically non-constrained articulation at the DRUJ, subject to dorsal-palmar translational instability [8] (Figure 2). Because of this bony incongruity, stability of the DRUJ is dependent on extracapsular (extrinsic) as well as intracapsular (intrinsic) structures. Principal extrinsic stabilizers are (1) dynamic tension of the extensor carpi ulnaris (ECU), (2) the semi-rigid 6th dorsal extensor compartment itself, (3) dynamic support by the pronator quadrates, and (4) the interosseous ligament of the forearm [9-12]. These extrinsic structures, however, play minor biomechanical roles in rotational forearm stability, compared with the TFCC as intrinsic structures of the radioulnar components. Previous anatomical and biomechanical studies have enabled us to understand how dc-TFCC is critical to the stability of the DRUJ [8,13,14].

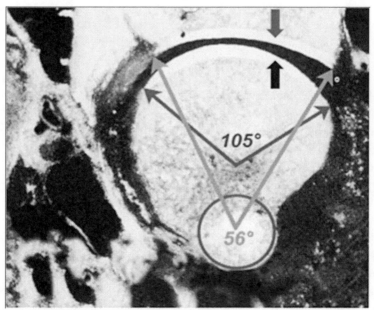

(Reprinted with permission [8]) .

Figure 2. Axial section through the radioulnar joint. While a black arrow indicates curvature of the seat of the ulna, a red arrow suggests curvature of the sigmoid notch. The obtuse angle of attack of the dc-TFCC (blue arrow) is oriented to prevent DRUJ subluxation. A green arrow indicates the sc-TFCC.

The following 2 anatomic factors are responsible for more a significant stabilizing effect of the dc-TFCC on the DRUJ stability than the sc-TFCC. First, most of the hyaline cartilage-covered distal end of the ulna has herniated against the dorsal DRUJ capsule, out from under the cover of the dorsal sc-TFCC in maximum pronation [15]. DRUJ stability in full pronation mainly depends on the restraining, pulling action of the palmar dc-TFCC, preventing excessive translation from occurring. Second, the obtuse angle of attack of the dc-TFCC is oriented to prevent DRUJ subluxation (Figure 2). Therefore, tears of the dc-TFCC lead to DRUJ instability and to symptomatic conditions of the wrist, such as ulnar-sided wrist pain. Surgical reattachment of avulsions of the dc-TFCC must be considered to provide stability for the DRUJ.

OPEN TECHNIQUES FOR THE TREATMENT OF AVULSED DC-TFCC FROM THE ULNAR FOVEA

Several authors recommend arthroscopic partial resection of the TFCC for relief of wrist pain [16,17]. However, the partial resection does not improve the biomechanical effect of the TFCC on DRUJ stability. Consequently, TFCC repair or reconstruction is advocated for cases of TFCC tear with DRUJ instability. Various arthroscopic techniques have been performed to suture the torn TFCC to the ulnocarpal space capsule and the ECU tendon subsheath [5,6,18-25]. These techniques can provide tension or tautness of the TFCC by direct suture of the TFC superficial portion. Although this leads to the relief of symptoms, such arthroscopic techniques do not improve the symptoms and provide DRUJ stability for cases with avulsed dc-TFCC from the ulnar fovea. Well-vascularized fibers, including the superficial radioulnar fibers inserting on the ulnar styloid and the deep fibers inserting onto the fovea, of the TFCC anchor the radius to the ulna along both its dorsal and palmar margins. Therefore, the dc-TFCC has healing potential at the site of reattachment by surgical procedures.

Open techniques for reattaching the dc-TFCC to its foveal insertion have been reported for cases with avulsed dc-TFCC from the ulnar fovea [5,8,26-30]. Nakamura et al. [29] introduced a 3-dimensional mattress suture of the disrupted TFCC for such cases. They reported that 36 of 37 patients (97%) achieved excellent or good results following their open procedure. Chou et al. [30] reported an open repair of avulsed TFCC utilizing a single suture anchor placed in the ulnar fovea. They demonstrated that the Modified Mayo Wrist

Score averaged 88 after this mini-open technique. All patients were rated as excellent or good at follow-up. Sennwald et al. [31] presented a reattachment of the avulsed TFCC to the ulnar fovea combined with an intra-articular shortening osteotomy of the ulnar head. They concluded that this technique gave the reduction of wrist pain without significant limitation of forearm rotation.

INDICATIONS AND CONTRAINDICATIONS FOR ARTHROSCOPIC REPAIR OF AVULSED DC-TFCC FROM THE ULNAR FOVEA

The author's diagnostic criteria for avulsion of the dc-TFCC from the ulnar fovea include (1) positive ulnar fovea sign [32], (2) positive provocative manners described by Kleinman [8], (3) DRUJ instability [32], and (4) MR image findings showing an area of high-signal-intensity at just distal to the fovea (Figure 3).

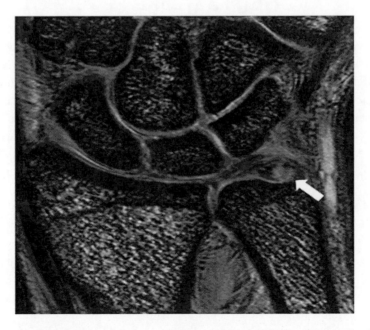

Figure 3. An MR coronal image shows an area of high-signal-intensity just distal to the ulnar fovea, suggesting avulsion of the dc-TFCC from the fovea.

The DRUJ instability is defined as an asymmetry of the constraint of the radius translation relative to the distal ulna in forearm pronation and supination [32]. Patients showing these findings apply a wrist brace to rest the affected wrist for 3 months. The patients without pain relief are indicated to scopic TFCC repair.

The contraindications to arthroscopic repair of avulsed dc-TFCC are as follows: (1) plain radiographs showing positive ulnar variance, (2) radiographic findings indicating arthritis of the radiocarpal joint and/or the DRUJ, and (3) arthroscopic findings showing degenerative changes (Class II) of the TFCC according to Palmer's classification [16]. For the positive ulnar variance wrist, ulnar shortening osteotomy has been recommended to reduce the load across the ulnocarpal space [33,34]. This procedure also stabilizes the DRUJ by increasing intrastructual tension of the TFCC [35]. However, in the case of avulsed dc-TFCC from the ulnar fovea, DRUJ stability is not achieved by the ulnar shortening osteotomy. Surgeons should keep in mind that the efficacy of ulnar shortening may be limited in such cases.

DRUJ ARTHROSCOPY

Previous reports recommended DRUJ arthroscopy as a reliable tool to identify dc-TFCC avulsion [5,6]. Because the DRUJ is a very small and tight jont, DRUJ arthroscopy is difficult and is not always possible. Without DRUJ instability, this joint cannot provide enough working space for a scope and instruments. On the other hand, when the dc-TFCC is injured, an arthroscope is easily introduced into the DRUJ and more working space is achieved for DRUJ exploration. The DRUJ is explored through the DRUJ portal with the forearm supinated to relax the dorsal capsule. An arthroscope is introduced dorsally between the 4th and 5th extensor compartments proximal to the sigmoid notch of the radius (DRUJ portal) underneath the TFCC. In smaller wrists, a volar ulnar portal, which is the interval between the flexor carpi ulnaris (FCU) and common flexor tendons, may be used. Degenerative changes in the articular surface of the sigmoid notch and the ulnar head are assessed. Loose bodies are occasionally found in the proximal space of the DRUJ. Synovitis is prevalent in the case of inflammatory arthritis. A DRUJ arthroscopy indicates the laceration or avulsion of the dc-TFCC from the ulnar fovea. Arthroscopic reattachment of the avulsed dc-TFCC to the ulnar fovea requires the radiocarpal portal to access to the TFCC surface.

ARTHROSCOPIC TECHNIQUES
FOR THE TREATMENT OF AVULSED
DC-TFCC FROM THE ULNAR FOVEA

Although previous reports have shown acceptable clinical outcomes following open techniques [26,29,30], a cautious and extensive exposure of the DRUJ and ulnocarpal space is required to reattach the avulsed dc-TFCC with bone anchors or intraosseous sutures [28-30]. The extensive joint exposure has potential to cause injury and destruction of surrounding structures, and a decrease in post-operative wrist and forearm ROM. Arthroscopic repair is a less invasive technique that could prevent such complications. However, techniques for arthroscopic repair of the avulsed dc-TFCC from the ulnar fovea have not been established because of technical difficulties. Traditional arthroscopic suture techniques may be of limited efficacy to provide DRUJ stability because they fail to reattach the avulsed dc-TFCC.

To date, there have been few arthroscopic techniques for the repair of the avulsed dc-TFCC [5,6,36]. Atzei et al. [5,6] reported an arthroscopic reattachment technique of the avulsed ac-TFCC onto the ulnar head using a suture anchor or screw system. First, avulsion of the dc-TFCC from the ulnar fovea is diagnosed by radiocarpal and DRUJ arthroscopy. Then, a screw or anchor with a pair of sutures is inserted to the foveal region. Once the screw or anchor is in place, the avulsed dc-TFCC is anchored to the ulnar fovea by an outside-in fashion of the repair sutures. At a mean follow-up of 18 months, 18 of 19 patients scored excellent and good according to the Modified Mayo Wrist Score.

AUTHOR'S PREFERRED
ARTHROSCOPIC TECHNIQUE [36]

Arthroscopic procedures are performed under general anesthesia with a pneumatic tourniquet. The patient is supine on the operating table. The shoulder is abducted 90° and the elbow is flexed 90°. The forearm is suspended vertically by a traction tower (CONMED, Lorgo, FL). 3.2 to 4.5 kg of traction is applied to all the fingers except for the thumb using Chinese finger traps (Figure 4). An 18-gauge needle is inserted first through the 6-U portal, which is on the ulnar side of the ECU tendon. Then, a 5 to 10 ml of saline solution is injected into the joint cavity. The inserted needle remains to use as an outflow. A 1.9 mm or 2.3 mm 30° arthroscope is introduced into the 3-4 portal, which is situated between the 3rd and 4th extensor compartments, using the standard technique. The 3-4 portal is established in the soft spot approximately 1 cm distal to Lister's tubercle. A small longitudinal skin incision is made with a No.15 scalpel blade. A blunt trocar is then introduced and angled 10° volar to be parallel to the articular surface of the distal radius. An accessory portal includes the 6-R or 4-5 portal. While the 6-R is on the radial side of the ECU tendon, the 4-5 portal is situated between the 4th and 5th extensor compartments. The lunotriquetral interosseous ligament, the scapholunate interosseous ligament, and the TFCC are each inspected for wear or tear.

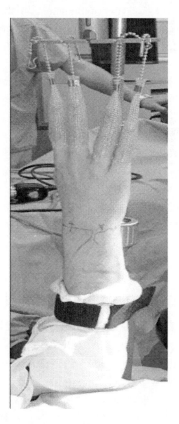

Figure 4. The forearm is suspended vertically by a traction tower. 3.2 to 4.5 kg of traction is applied to all the fingers except for the thumb using Chinese finger traps.

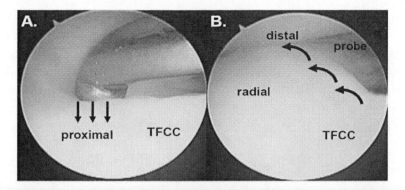

Figure 5. A. A loss of the normal trampoline effect. B. A displacement of the TFCC distally and radially to the center of the radiocarpal joint (positive hook test).

The articular surfaces of the lunate, the triquetrum and the distal radius are also investigated. After investigating the conditions of the TFCC surface, TFCC resilience (trampoline effect) on ballottement and radial mobility of the ulnar-most border of the TFCC (hook test) are confirmed using a probe to make a diagnosis [5,6,31]. The final diagnosis of avulsed dc-TFCC from the ulnar fovea is determined by a loss of the normal trampoline effect (Figure 5A) and a displacement of the TFCC distally and radially to the center of the radiocarpal joint (positive hook test) (Figure 5B) by each manner described above [5,6,31,36]. The author thinks that a combination of pre-operative physical and MRI findings with radiocarpal arthroscopic observation provides a diagnosis of dc-TFCC avulsion from the ulnar fovea. Therefore, the observation by DRUJ arthroscopy is not performed to identify the dc-TFCC avulsion.

Once the diagnosis has been confirmed, a 1.5 cm longitudinal incision is made around the ulnar neck and the ulna is exposed between the ECU and the FCU tendon. A 1.5-mm Kirschner wire used as a guide pin is inserted from the ulnar neck to the foveal region of the ulnar head under C-arm visualization (Figure 6). An original guiding device is used to confirm the anatomical position of the inserted Kirschner wire. Over the inserted wire, a 2.9 mm cannulated drill is driven to create an osseous tunnel 2.9 mm in diameter from the ulnar neck to the foveal surface. This procedure simultaneously debrides fibrous connective tissues at the foveal surface (Figure 7A). Under arthroscopic guidance, a 2-0 non-absorbable suture (Prolene, ETHICON, Some Ville, NJ or FiberWire, Arthrex, Naples, FL) passed into a 21 gauge needle is placed into the TFCC through the osseous tunnel. Then, a 3-0 non-absorbable suture loop is advanced into the TFCC using the same manner. The suture end is captured by the loop and delivered out of the osseous tunnel by proximally withdrawing the loop (Figure 7B). Then, the two free ends of the repair suture are pulled through the osseous tunnel to bring the suture onto the TFCC surface. The avulsed TFCC is anchored to the fovea in this manner. Near-normal tension of the TFCC is then reconstituted by tightening both ends of the suture. With the forearm in neutral rotation, the suture is tied onto the ulnar periosteum over the proximal entrance of the osseous tunnel (Figure 7C).

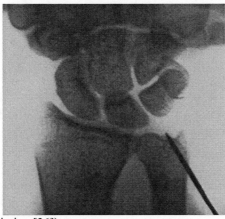

(Reprinted with permission [36])

Figure 6. Under C-arm visualization, a Kirschner wire used as a guide pin is inserted from the ulnar neck to the ulnar fovea.

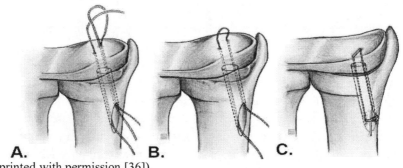

(Reprinted with permission [36]).

Figure 7. A. An osseous tunnel from the ulnar neck to the ulnar fovea. Using a suture loop, the end of repair suture is delivered out of the osseous tunnel. B. The 2 free ends of the suture are pulled through the osseous tunnel to bring the suture onto the TFCC surface. C. The avulsed TFCC is anchored to the fovea with near normal tension. The suture is tied on to the ulnar periosteum.

To protect the repaired TFCC from forearm rotation, each patient is splinted with a long-arm cast in 45-60° of supination for 4 weeks post-operatively. Then, a removable wrist brace is applied for an additional 2 weeks. At 6 weeks after operation, we direct the patients to begin vigorous rehabilitation of the wrist and forearm.

COMPLICATIONS

Complications associated with wrist arthroscopy are relatively infrequent. However, surgeons should understand the risks of associated complications in performing wrist arthroscopy and practice arthroscopic techniques to prevent them. Complications can be considered in the following 3 categories: 1) complications related to specific tissues around the wrist joint, 2) complications related to execution of the procedure, and 3) complications related to final post-operative results [37].

1. Complications Related to Specific Tissues around the Wrist Joint

Any of the intra- and extra-articular tissues around the wrist can be injured during the course of arthroscopic procedures. To prevent tissue injuries, instruments should be introduced and manipulated in a gentle fashion. In addition, the surgeons must notice any resistance or impediment to the movement of instruments in the joint cavity. When resistance is encountered, the surgeons must stop the movement of instruments and decipher the cause.

The extensor tendons except for the extensor indicis proprius and the extensor digiti minimi are usually palpable. Generally, tendon injury by the insertion of instruments is avoided if the surgeons pay attention to the anatomy related to the portals, palpating and marking the location of each tendon compartment. Avoiding deep incisions with the scalpel and applying blunt trocars prevent any injury to tendons. In performing TFCC repair using outside-in techniques, suture knots tied to the capsule or the floor of the 6th extensor compartment often irritate the ECU tendon. This complication is accentuated by using monofilament sutures.

The most serious complication during arthroscopic TFCC repairs is injury to the dorsal sensory branch of the ulnar nerve (DSUBN). The incidence of this neurological injury resulting from wrist arthroscopic procedures ranged from less than 0.1% to 2% ... Most of the DSUBN injuries are transient neurapraxia that recover spontaneously within 3 to 4 months [6]. Understanding the course and patterns of arborization of the DSUBN is critical to minimize the risk of this nerve injury during wrist arthroscopic procedures. Spreading the soft tissue with a fine-point hemostat prior to instrument insertion enables the nerve to move away from instruments. This approach, and incising skin only, seems to be the most effective means to prevent the DSUBN injury during wrist arthroscopy.

One of the most considerable complications in performing arthroscopic surgeries is injury to articular cartilage by the introduced arthroscope and accessory instruments into the joint. The risk of this complication increases in small joints, such as the wrist. Improperly placed portals do not lead the instruments into the appropriate place. Misled portals may easily puncture and lacerate articular cartilage. It must be noted that hyaline cartilage injury is never naturally healed and results in osteoarthritis.

The condition of the patient's skin should be carefully considered during surgery. The application of finger traps damages finger skin, especially in the presence of predisposing systemic conditions including rheumatoid arthritis, systemic lupus, and senile atrophy. In such cases, finger traps should be placed on all of the fingers except for the thumb. The least strenous traction force should be applied to the fingers.

2. Complications Related to Performing Wrist Arthroscopic Procedures

In performing any surgical procedure, complications that impede execution of the procedure can occur. These complications may have temporal or lasting effects on operated hands.

Intra-articular bleeding in performing wrist arthroscopy obscures the visual field. Bleeding in the wrist joint can occur from lacerations of the capsule or synovial tissues. If bleeding is uncontrollable, complete fluid exchange is required. The use of radiofrequency probes is effective in preventing bleeding, especially from synovial tissues.

An imbalance in the inflow and outflow of irrigating solutions introduces bubbles into the joint. This can compromise visibility for arthroscopic procedures. In addition, surgeons should pay attention to the occurrence of edema due to extravasation of the irrigating fluid into subcutaneous tissue. This may lead to compartment syndrome or joint stiffness after surgery. Dry techniques for joint exploration are advocated to reduce soft tissue infiltration and swelling [38].

The use of radiofrequency (RF) devices has increased in arthroscopic TFCC debridement, synovectomy, scapholunate ligament thermal shrinkage [39-41]. Recently, thermal capsulorrhaphy for carpal instability has also been performed [42]. The RF probes used in wrist arthroscopy raise joint fluid temperature, increasing the risk of thermal damage to tissues around the wrist joint. A previous study reported that among 47 patients who underwent wrist arthroscopy with thermal ablation, 4 sustained serious complications including tendon ruptures and a full-thickness skin burn; thus, there was a 9% complication rate [43]. An experimental study showed that maximum joint temperature using an RF probe was greater than 60°C in no-outflow conditions. Such a temperature has the potential to damage adjacent tissues [44]. On the other hand, the use of an outlet portal reduced the joint temperature. Maintaining adequate outflow is useful to prevent thermal damage to tissues when using RF probes during wrist arthroscopy.

3. Complications Affecting Ultimate Post-operative Results

The development of post-operative superficial or deep infection and complex regional pain syndrome (CRPS) are serious complications potentially affecting post-operative results. Although the occurrence of these complications is not frequent in wrist arthroscopy, these complications lead to the impairment of wrist function. Infections are usually prevented by a prophylactic dose of parenteral antibiotics before initiating the surgery. However, surgeons should make an early diagnosis of these complications and start appropriate treatment as soon as possible.

REFERENCES

[1]   Takagi, K. (1982). The classic. Arthroscope. Kenji Takagi. J. Jap. Orthop. Assoc., 1939. *Clin. Orthop. Relat. Res.*, 167, 6-8.

[2]   Whipple, TL; Marotta, J; Powell, J. (1986). Techniques of wrist arthroscopy. *Arthroscopy*, 2, 244-252.

[3]   Palmer, AK; Werner, FW. (1981). The triangular fibrocartilage complex of the wrist–anatomy and function. *J. Hand Surg.*, 6, 153-162.

[4]   Nakamura, T; Yabe, Y; Horiuchi, Y. (1996). Functional anatomy of the triangular fibrocartilage complex. *J. Hand Surg. Br.*, 21, 581-586.

[5]   Atzei,,A. (2009). New trends in arthroscopic management of type 1-B TFCC injuries with DRUJ instability. *J. Hand Surg. Er.,* 34, 582-591.

[6]   Atzei, A; Rizzo, A; Luchetti, R; Fairplay, T. (2008). Arthroscopic foveal repair of triangular fibrocartilage complex peripheral lesion with distal radioulnar joint instability. *Tech. Hand Up Extrem. Surg.*, 12, 226-235.

[7]   Nakamura, T; Makita, A. (2000). The proximal ligamentous component of the triangular fibrocartilage complex: functional anatomy and three-dimensional changes in length of the radioulnar ligament during pronation-supination. *J. Hand Surg. Br.*, 25, 479-486.

[8]   Kleinman, WB. (2007). Stability of the distal radioulnar joint: Biomechanics, pathophysiology, physical diagnosis, and restoration of function: what we have learned in 25 years. *J. Hand Surg. Am.,* 32, 1086-1106.

[9]   Goldner, JL; Hayes, MG. (1979). Stabilization of the remaining ulna using one-half of the extensor carpi ulnaris tendon after re-section of the distal ulna. *Orthop. Trans.*, 3, 330-331.

[10] Hotchkiss, RN; An, KN; Sowa, DT; Basta, S; Weiland, AJ. (1989). An anatomic and mechanical study of the interosseous membrane of the forearm: pathomechanics of the proximal migration of the radius. *J. Hand Surg. Am.,* 14, 256-261.

[11] Spinner, M; Kaplan, EB. (1970). Extensor carpi ulnaris: its relationship to stability of the distal radio-ulnar joint. *Clin. Orthop. Relat. Res.*, 68, 124-128.

[12] Ruby, LK; Ferenz, CC; Dell, PC. (1996). The pronator quadrates interposition transfer: an adjunct to re-section arthroplasty of the distal radioulnar joint. *J. Hand Surg. Am.*, 21, 60-65.

[13] Af Ekenstam, F; Hagert, CG. (1985). Anatomical studies on the geometry and stability of the distal radioulnar joint. *Scand. J. Plast. Reconstr. Surg.,* 19, 17-25.

[14] Haugstvedt, JR; Berger, RA; Nakamura, T; Neale, P; Berglund, L; An, KN. (2006). Relative contributions of the ulnar attachments of the triangular fibrocartilage complex to the dynamic stability of the distal radioulnar joint. *J. Hand Surg. Am.*, 31, 445-451.

[15] Kleinman, WB; Graham, TJ. (1998). The distal radioulnar joint capsule: clinical anatomy and role in post-traumatic limitation of forearm rotation. *J. Hand Surg. Am.*, 23, 588-599.

[16] Palmer, AK. (1989). Triangular fibrocartilage complex lesions: a classification. *J. Hand Surg. Am.*, 14, 594-606.

[17] Menon, J; Wood, VE; Schoene, HR; et al. (1984). Isolated tears of the triangular fibrocartilage of the wrist: results of partial excision. *J. Hand Surg. Am.,* 9, 527-530.

[18] Badia, A; Jimènez, A. (2006). Arthroscopic repair of peripheral triangular fibrocartilage complex tears with suture welding: a technical report. *J. Hand Surg. Am.*, 31, 1303-1307.

[19] Bohringer, G; Schadel-Hopfner, M; Petermann, J; Gotzen, L. (2002). A method for all-inside arthroscopic repair of Palmer 1B triangular fibrocartilage complex tears. *Arthroscopy*, 18, 211-213.

[20] Conca, M; Conca, R; Pria, AD. (2004). Preliminary experience of fully arthroscopic repair of triangular fibrocartulage complex lesions. *Arthroscopy,* 20, 79-82.

[21] Corso, SJ; Savoie, FH; Geissler, WB; Whipple, TL; Jiminez, W; Jenkins, N. (1997). Arthroscopic repair of peripheral avulsions of the triangular fibrocartilage complex of the wrist: a multi-center study. *Arthroscopy,* 13, 78-84.

[22] Haugstvedt, JR; Husby, T. (1999). Results of repair of peripheral tears in the triangular fibrocartilage complex using an arthroscopic suture technique. *Scand. J. Plast. Reconstr. Surg. Hand Surg.*, 33, 439-447.

[23] Trumble, TE; Gilbert, M; Vedder, N. (1997). Isolated tears of the triangular fibrocartilage: management by early arthroscopic repair. *J. Hand Surg. Am.*, 22, 57-65.

[24] Whipple, TL; Geissler, WB. (1993). Arthroscopic management of wrist triangular fibrocartilage complex injuries in the athlete. *Orthopedics*, 16, 1061-1067.

[25] Zachee, B; De Smet, L; Fabry, G. (1993). Arthroscopic suturing of TFCC lesions. *Arthroscopy*, 9, 242-243.

[26] Bain, GI; Roth, JH. (2007). Surgical approaches to the distal radioulnar joint. *Tech. Hand Up Extrem. Surg.*, 11, 51-56.

[27] Garcia-Elias, M; Smith, DE; Llusa, M. (2003). Surgical approach to the triangular fibrocartilage complex. *Tech. Hand Up Extrem. Surg.*, 7, 134-140.

[28] Hermansdorfer, JD; Kleinman, WB. (1991). Management of chronic peripheral tears of the triangular fibrocartilage complex. *J. Hand Surg. Am.*, 16, 340-346.

[29] Nakamura, T; Nakao, Y; Ikegami, H; Sato, K; Takayama, S. (2004). Open repair of the ulnar disruption of the triangular fibrocartilage complex with double three-dimensional mattress suturing technique. *Tech. Hand Up Extrem. Surg.*, 8, 116-123.

[30] Chou, KH; Sarris, IK; Soteteanos, DG. (2003). Suture anchor repair of ulnar-sided triangular fibrocartilage complex tears. *J. Hand Surg. Br.*, 28, 546-550.

[31] Sennwald, GR; Lauterburg, M; Zdravkovic, V. (1995). A new technique of reattachment after traumatic avulsion of the TFCC at its ulnar insertion. *J. Hand Surg. Br.*, 20, 178-184.

[32] Tay, SC; Tomita, K; Berger, RA. (2007). The "ulnar fovea sign" for defining ulnar wrist pain: an analysis of sensitivity and specificity. *J. Hand Surg. Am.*, 32, 438-444.

[33] Iwasaki, N; Ishikawa, J; Kato, H; Minam, M; Minami, A. (2007). Factors affecting results of ulnar shortening for ulnar impaction syndrome. *Clin. Orthop. Relat. Res.*, 465, 215-219.

[34] Minami, A; Kato, H. (1984). Ulnar shortening for triangular fibrocartilage complex of the wrist: results of partial resection. *J. Hand Surg. Am.*, 9, 527-530.

[35] Nishikawa, M; Nakamura, T; Nakao, Y; Nagura, T; Yoyama, Y. (2005). Ulnar shortening effect on distal radioulnar stability: a biomechanical study. *J. Hand Surg. Am.*, 30, 719-726.

[36] Iwasaki, N; Minami, A. (2009). Arthroscopically-assisted reattachment of avulsed triangular fibrocartilage complex to the fovea of the ulnar head. *J. Hand Surg. Am.*, 34, 1323-1326.

[37] Whipple, TL. (1992). *Arthroscopic Surgery: The Wrist. Philadelphia*, PA:J.B. Lippincott Company.

[38] Del Pinal, F; Garcia-Bernal, FJ; Pisani, D; et al. (2007). Dry arthroscopy of the wrist: surgical technique. *J. Hand Surg. Am.*, 32, 119-123.

[39] Darlis, NA; Weiser, RW; Sotereanos, DG. (2005). Arthroscopic triangular fibrocartilage complex debridement using radiofrequency probes. *J. Hand Surg. Br.*, 30, 638-642.

[40] Darlis, NA; Weiser, RW; Sotereanos, DG. (2005). Partial scapholunate ligament injuries treated with arthroscopic debridement and thermal shrinkage. *J. Hand Surg. Am.*, 30, 908-914.

[41] DeWal, H; Ahn, A; Raskin, KB. (2002). Thermal energy in arthroscopic surgery of the wrist. *Clin. Sports Med.,* 21, 727-753.

[42] Mason, WT; Hargreaves, DG. (2007). Arthroscopic thermal capsulorrhaphy for palmar mid-carpal instability. *J. Hand Surg. Br.,* 32, 411-416.

[43] Pell, RF IV; Uhl, RL. (2004). Complications of thermal ablation in wrist arthroscopy. *Arthroscopy,* 20(Suppl 2), 84-86.

[44] Sotereanos, DG; Darlis, NA; Kokkalis, ZT; Zanaros, G; Altman, GT; Miller, MC. (2009). Effects of radiofrequency probe application on irrigation fluid temperature in the wrist joint. *J. Hand Surg. Am.,* 34, 1832-1837.

In: Arthroscopy
Editors: K. Elani et al.

ISBN: 978-1-61470-955-8
© 2012 Nova Science Publishers, Inc.

Chapter V

Use of a Single Intra-Articular Injection of Sodium Hyaluronate as a Complement to Arthroscopic Lysis and Lavage in Wilkes Stage III and IV Disease

Miguel-Angel Morey-Mas,[1]* Luisa Varela-Sende,[2] Aitor García-Sánchez, [3] Jorge Caubet-Biayna,[4] and José-Ignacio Iriarte-Ortabe[5]

[1]Staff Surgeon, Assistant Professor of Oral and Maxillofacial Surgery
[2]Head of Pharmacology, Qualified Person of Pharmacovigilance
Department of Clinical Pharmacovigilance, Masterfarm
Laboratories, Barcelona, Spain
[3]Resident of Oral and Maxillofacial Surgery
[4]Staff Surgeon, Assistant Professor of Oral and Maxillofacial Surgery
[5]Head, Assistant Professor of Oral and Maxillofacial Surgery
Department of Oral and Maxillofacial Surgery, Son Dureta
University Hospital, Palma de Mallorca, Spain

* Correspondence to: Miguel-Angel Morey-Mas. C/ Albo, 15 principal A, 07013 Palma Mallorca,
Spain. Tel.: 0034 629344416. E-mail: mmoreym@gmail.com.

ABSTRACT

Purpose: To evaluate the analgesic efficacy and function after a single intra-articular (i.a.) injection of sodium hyaluronate (SH) (1 ml at 1%) into temporomandibular joint (TMJ) as a complement to arthroscopic lysis and lavage in Wilkes stage III and IV disease.

Patients and Methods: A comparative, randomized, double-blind, pilot controlled clinical trial was performed. Forty patients with an internal disorder of the TMJ (Wilkes III-IV) with joint pain and/or mouth-opening limitation were randomly assigned to 2 groups of 20. The experimental group received Ringer lactate plus an injection of 1 ml of SH in the superior joint space of the TMJ after arthroscopy, whereas the control group was given Ringer lactate without viscoelastic supplementation during arthroscopy. Clinical evaluation was carried out using a visual analogue scale (VAS) on the pain and joint function criteria. A secondary evaluation examined disc position and tolerance of treatment. The patients were followed up for 6 months with five assessments. Suitable parametric and nonparametric statistic tests were performed, and the level of statistical significance was set at .05.

Results: The reduction in joint pain was statistically significant in the treatment group with respect to the control group on the visits on days 14 and 84. Compared to baseline, the level of analgesia was statistically significant in the treated group on day 28. The tolerance of treatment was considered optimal in the control and experimental groups.

Conclusion: An i.a. injection of SH following arthroscopic lysis and lavage is effective in reducing pain in patients with TMJ dysfunction. Furthermore, SH enhances post-surgical recovery. The analgesic effect of treatment with SH is maintained in the long term.

INTRODUCTION

Several lines of treatment have been described in the literature for TMJ dysfunction including surgery, [1,2] physiotherapy, [3] occlusal splint therapy, [4] arthrocentesis [5] and arthroscopy. [6] Lysis and lavage with arthroscopy has shown its efficacy as a method for diagnosis and treatment. It improves the symptoms and restores jaw function in patients with TMJ dysfunction by removing the catabolites of the inflammatory processes and loosening the adhesions thanks to the pressure of the lavage fluid. [7,8,9]

Some studies showed the efficacy of i.a. injection with SH in treating disc displacement with or without reduction, [10] administered either once only

[11] or repeatedly, [12,13] either alone [14] or following arthrocentesis. [15] These series generally compare the efficacy of i.a. infiltration of SH with corticosteroids, [16] placebo, [10] placement of a splint [17] or an orally-administered drug. [11] Although different authors referred indirectly to the use of SH in their arthroscopic surgery procedures, [18,19] there is no study that specifically analyzes the use of this product as a complement to arthroscopy. The use of an i.a. injection of SH when compared to a Ringer solution may help in the arthroscopic recovery due to the restoration of the protective action of the endogenous hyaluronic acid eliminated during arthroscopic procedure.

The aim of our study was to evaluate the post-surgical benefit in terms of pain reduction and joint function improvement of a single i.a. injection of SH (1 ml at 1%) compared to a Ringer solution as a complement to arthroscopic lysis and lavage in patients with Wilkes stage III and IV disease.

PATIENTS AND METHODS

A comparative, randomized, single-center (Hospital Son Dureta, Palma de Mallorca, Spain), double-blind study was designed. Fifty one patients were registered. Eleven patients were not randomized because they were not surgical candidates according to clinical criteria. Forty patients were randomly distributed into 2 groups of 20. The experimental group was administered a 1 ml injection of SH (Ostenil® mini, Masterfarm Laboratories, Barcelona, Spain) in the superior joint space of the TMJ, following arthroscopic lysis and lavage (treatment group). The control group was given i.a. Ringer lactate during arthroscopic lysis and lavage without final viscoelastic supplementation (control group). To ensure that it was a double-blind study, the surgical procedure was carried out by the main investigator, whereas the later evolutions were performed by another investigator not associated in any way with the surgical process.

A follow-up of all the patients during 6 months was carried out, exempting a patient who was not assessable due to the lack of magnetic resonance image (MRI) after arthroscopy. Men and female patients aged over 18 years with magnetic resonance imaging-confirmed disc displacement with or without reduction and Wilkes stages III and IV TMJ disorder were included. The study protocol required patients to have TMJ joint pain and/or mouth-opening limitation (TMJ pain at rest or mastication of over 20 mm on the visual analogue scale and/or maximum jaw opening of 30 mm or less). It was also necessary the absence of response to conservative measures (surgical splint, medication, physiotherapy), for at least 6 months. Major exclusion criteria included degenerative illnesses such as rheumatoid arthritis; arthrocentesis, arthroscopy or previous open surgery on the same joint; extra-articular pain; impossibility of correct performing of the arthroscopic technique and severe osteoarthritis or disc perforation (Wilkes V).

TMJ arthroscopy was performed under general anesthesia and nasotracheal intubation. The technique began by expanding the superior joint space with an injection of 4 cc of saline solution and Bupivacaine 0.5% in equal proportions, using a 23 G needle. The superior joint space was then carefully punctured with straight and curved-end trocars to insert a cannula, and its position checked using a Dyonics 1.9 mm diameter, 30° angular arthroscope (Smith and Nephew, Melbourne, Australia). A continuous Ringer lactate irrigation system was connected. Once drainage had been established and after inspecting the superior joint space, a second cannula was inserted using the triangulation technique at an anterior-superior angle, which was manipulated to move the disc and release any adhesions. Meanwhile lavage continued with at least 200 cc of Ringer solution. This second portal was finally used to administer 1 ml of SH in the treatment group, and its entry in the superior joint space was visually confirmed arthroscopically.

The primary efficacy parameter was analgesic activity, measured with a 100 mm VAS. Further evaluation of TMJ function was made in terms of maximum interincisal opening (in mm), deviation of the jaw from the midline when opening, protrusion and lateral movements and crepitus or grating in the joints. The secondary efficacy parameters were the disc position evaluated by magnetic resonance imaging (MRI) and overall evaluation by the patient and the investigator on a 5-point scale from worse (0) to optimal (4). Adverse effects were also noted. The patients were evaluated at the beginning of the study (7 days before arthroscopy), on the day of the intervention (day 0) and on days 14, 28, 56, 84 and 168. The visit before arthroscopy (-7 days pre-surgical) was considered the baseline for the objective and clinical measures, and the visit on day 14 was considered a baseline for the comparative analyses in percentage of patients with pain improvement. From day 14 on, we considered the groups homogeneous and comparable, since 2 weeks is the average time for post-surgical recovery (in both cases pain was due to the surgery and not to the joint pathology itself). MRI evaluation of the disc position was made at the baseline visit and at the last visit (day 168). The study protocol was previously approved by the *Comité de Ensayos Clínicos de la Islas Baleares* - Spain [Balearic Islands Clinical Trials Committee]. All patients had to give their signed informed consent to be included in the protocol.

The results were statistically analyzed using SPSS statistical system version 15.0 (*SPSS* Inc, *Chicago*, *Illinois*). Suitable parametric and non-parametric tests were performed and statistical significance level set at 0.05.

RESULTS

40 patients were recruited and randomly divided into 2 groups. Follow-up was complete in all patients, so all of them reached the visit at six months (day 168). The average age of the patients was 35.3 years (SD=13.3) and 92.5% of them were women. There were no statistically significance differences between the groups (p>0.05).

Most of the patients evaluated in both groups presented disc displacement without reduction. Table 1 describes the disc position at the beginning and end of treatment: at the baseline visit, 79.5% of the study population presented a displaced disc without reduction, whereas by day 168, this parameter had decreased to 68.4%. No statistically significant differences were observed in disc position between the treatment and comparator groups (p>0.05).

Table 1. Progress of disc position at the beginning and end of treatment

	Treatment group		Comparator group		Overall		$p^{a,b}$
	n	%	n	%	n	%	
Baseline visit	19	100.0	20	100.0	39	100.0	-
Normal	0	0.0	0	0.0	0	0.0	
Displaced with reduction	3	15.8	5	25.0	8	20.5	0.4765
Displaced without reduction	16	84.2	15	75.0	31	79.5	
Visit day 168	18	100.0	20	100.0	38	100.0	-
Normal	2	11.1	3	15.0	5	13.2	
Displaced with reduction	3	16.7	4	20.0	7	18.4	0.8877
Displaced without reduction	13	72.2	13	65.0	26	68.4	

[a] Statistically significant results in boldface (p-value < 0.05).

[b] Chi-squared test.

Table 2. Differences in joint pain over time (VAS scale)

	Treatment group			Control group			Overall		
	Mean	Range	$p^{a,b}$	Mean	Range	$p^{a,b}$	Mean	Range	$p^{a,c}$
Baseline visit	62,0	31,0 - 100,0	-	47,9 (20,2)	18,0 - 90,0	-	54,8 (21,0)	18,0 - 100,0	-
Visit day 14	32,4	0,0 - 80,0	0,000 7	17,5 (16,7)	0,0 - 59,0	0,000 2	24,7 (21,5)	0,0 - 80,0	0,036 0
Visit day 28	20,3	0,0 - 69,0	0,000 2	15,2 (18,4)	0,0 - 56,0	0,000 2	17,7 (18,7)	0,0 - 69,0	0,305 8
Visit day 56	22,1	0,0 - 71,0	0,000 5	14,0 (19,7)	0,0 - 74,0	0,000 1	17,9 (21,7)	0,0 - 74,0	0,200 5
Visit day 84	23,0	0,0 - 61,0	0,000 2	10,9 (16,1)	0,0 - 62,0	0,000 1	16,8 (19,0)	0,0 - 62,0	0,042 0
Visit day 168	19,0	0,0 - 59,0	0,000 1	9,6 (17,0)	0,0 - 64,0	0,000 1	14,2 (19,4)	0,0 - 64,0	0,100 4

[a] Statistically significant results in boldface (p-value<0,05).
[b] Wilcoxon Test.
[c] U de Mann-Whitney Test.

In analyzing the primary endpoint (pain control), a patient was considered to have improved if each scale decreased by at least *10 mm* for each visit in comparison to baseline (-7 days pre-surgical). Statistically significant differences (p<0.05) were seen between the treatment group and the comparator group in joint pain on day 14 and day 84 (Table 2). Statistically significant differences (p<0.05) can also be seen in both the treatment and comparator groups, comparing joint pain at the first visit and at the rest of the visits (significant reduction).

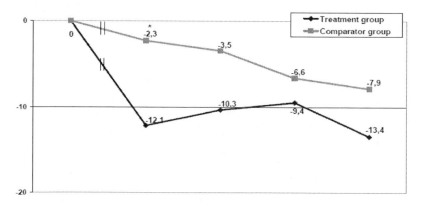

Figure 1. Differences in TMJ pain over time (VAS scale), taking day 14 as baseline.

Figure 1 shows the variation in the differences in TMJ pain (taking day 14 as baseline), both in the group treated with SH injection following arthroscopic lysis and lavage and in the control group which received arthroscopy and lavage with Ringer lactate without final viscoelastic supplementation. These changes were greatest, and statistically significant, for the treatment group on day 28.

Additionally, the percentage of patients in whom the joint pain scale score (VAS scale) decreased by at least *10 mm* compared to day 14 was calculated. A significant increase was observed in the percentage of patients in the comparator group who improved throughout the study (Friedman; $p<0.05$). Moreover, for each visit, more than 45% of the patients in the treatment group and more than 20% in the comparator group improved. Statistically significant differences were seen between groups on days 28 and 168 in the percentage of patients with pain improvement compared to day 14 (Chi-squared; $p<0.05$) (Figure 2).

The maximum interincisal opening was also evaluated at each visit, from the baseline visit to the visit on day 168. No statistically significant differences were observed in maximum mouth opening between the treatment and control groups ($p>0.05$). Statistically significant differences were found in the treatment group ($p<0.05$) in the maximum mouth opening between the baseline and day 56 visits, and between the baseline and day 168 visits, and also both in the control group and the overall population between the baseline visit and days 28, 56, 84 and 168 (Table 3).

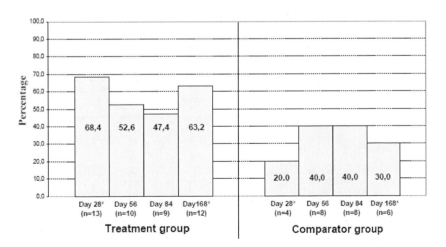

Figure 2. Percentage of patients whose joint pain improved by at least 10 mm compared to day 14.

Table 3. Changes in maximum mouth opening (mm)

	Treatment group			Comparator group		
	Mean (SD)	Range	$p^{a,b}$	Mean (SD)	Range	$p^{a,b}$
Baseline visit (TG=19 CG=20)	31.5 (12.1)	12.0 - 60.0	-	30.8 (9.8)	16.0 - 50.0	-
Visit day 14 (TG=18 CG=20)	29.6 (9.7)	10.0 - 58.0	0.2553	30.9 (5.7)	20.0 - 40.0	0.6284
Visit day 28 (TG=18 CG=20)	33.4 (8.5)	22.0 - 61.0	0.5561	34.4 (7.3)	26.0 - 50.0	**0.0089**
Visit day 56 (TG=17 CG=20)	36.1 (7.6)	27.0 - 61.0	**0.0435**	36.6 (8.1)	28.0 - 55.0	**0.0005**
Visit day 84 (TG=17 CG=19)	34.7 (8.4)	24.0 - 60.0	0.1544	36.7 (8.0)	25.0 - 55.0	**0.0005**
Visit day 168 (TG=19 CG=20)	36.8 (7.4)	27.0 - 60.0	**0.0150**	38.9 (6.8)	31.0 - 55.0	**0.0003**

[a] Statistically significant results in boldface (p-value <0.05); [b] Wilcoxon Test.

Treatment tolerance was analyzed from the point of view of both the patient and the investigator. On day 14, 60.5% of the overall population considered the treatment optimal or good, and on day 168, 74.3%. At the end of the study, a larger percentage of patients in the comparator group considered the therapy optimal compared to the treatment group, although the difference was not statistically significant (p>0.05).

Table 4. Safety and Tolerance

	Treatment group		Comparator group	
	n	$\%^{1}$	n	$\%^{1}$
Assessable patients for safety	20	100.0	20	100.0
Absence of adverse events	17	85.0	18	90.0
Presence of adverse events	3	15.0	2	10.0
Assessable patients for safety	20	100.0	20	100.0
No adverse event	17	85.0	18	90.0
One adverse event	2	10.0	2	10.0
Two adverse events	0	0.0	0	0.0
More than two adverse events	1	5.0	0	0.0

[1] Percentage calculated with respect to all assessable patients for safety.

With regard to adverse events, these occurred in 15.0% (n=3) of the patients in the treatment group, and 10% (n=2) in the comparator group (Table 4). The most common adverse events were earache and joint noise, each present in 5.0% (n=2) of the population. Tolerability both at the start and the end of the study was considered better in the control group (a larger percentage of patients qualifying tolerability of treatment as good or excellent) than in the treatment group, but the differences were not statistically significant.

CONCLUSION

A number of studies describe the results of arthroscopic lysis and lavage of the TMJ in the medium and long term, and high success rates are achieved in reducing pain and improving joint mobility, even in advanced states of dysfunction. [20,21,22,23,24,25] The most complete retrospective study demonstrating that arthroscopic surgery of the TMJ is a safe, beneficial and effective technique in treating temporomandibular dysfunction was carried out by McCain et al [1]. Murakami et al [26] published a 5-year follow-up study that correlated the diagnostic staging with the surgical procedure used. The cases in Wilkes stages III and IV were treated with lysis and lavage, whereas the patients in stage V were submitted to more advanced arthroscopic techniques. The success rates (in terms of jaw mobility, pain control and dietary habits) in stages III, IV and V were 86%, 92% ad 93% respectively, with no significant differences being found between the three groups. Most of the patients evaluated in our study in both groups presented disc displacement without reduction, to be expected as they were patients who had failed to respond to the previous conservative measures, corresponding to Wilkes stages III and IV. With respect to Wilkes stage V, some studies question the efficacy of the lysis and lavage (as in Murakami, in addition to Indresano [23] and McCain, [18] who recommend more complete arthroscopic operating techniques and arthrotomies for treating this advanced stage with disc perforation). In our study, we therefore decided to consider Wilkes stage V as a reason for exclusion.

Other studies support the efficacy of i.a. injection of SH in TMJ dysfunction treatment in different stages, used as a single treatment or with other drugs (glucocorticoids, analgesics, etc.) and other treatments (arthrocentesis, splint, etc.). [10-17] However, there is controversy over the use of SH as a complement to arthroscopic treatment of TMJ, and few references in the literature specifically analyze this question. [18,19,23]

The aim of our study was to evaluate the analgesic efficacy and TMJ function after a single i.a. injection of SH into temporomandibular joint as a complement to arthroscopic lysis and lavage in Wilkes stage III and IV disease. The results show that SH is effective in pain improvement and in the maximum interincisal opening. In addition SH maintains its analgesic effect over a period of at least 6 months.

Our study therefore differs from Guarda et al [17] and Alpaslan and Alpaslan, [15] in which arthrocentesis was performed with or without viscoelastic supplementation. It is necessary to separate the mechanisms of action of the two treatments (lysis and lavage and SH injection) and to attribute the therapeutic effect corresponding to each one. In joints with dysfunction, arthroscopy is responsible for the removal by lavage of catabolites of inflammation from the synovial fluid, and also for the lysis of adhesions, as a result of the increased hydrostatic pressure of the irrigation fluid (Ringer Lactate) in the joint space, and for the lysis of adhesions under direct view with instrumentation techniques. [27,28] This is what gives arthroscopy greater therapeutic potential than arthrocentesis, with which it is not possible to ensure the total removal of the adhesions and it is also not possible to categorically state that the lavage is correctly established in the i.a. space. SH has a lubricating, protective and repairing effect on the joint surfaces, as well as analgesic and anti-inflammatory action. [29,30] The analgesic effect is attributed to the blocking of nociceptive terminals and is directly proportional to the molecular weight of the SH [31] and the elastoviscosity of the solution. [32] Furthermore, the SH prevents the formation of adhesions, [33] which explains its long term beneficial effect. Our results match those of other studies in observing better pain control after 6 months, a time in which the exogenous SH has disappeared from the joint space.

In the processes of TMJ dysfunction, the concentration and molecular weight of the hyaluronic acid in the synovial fluid decrease as a result of the dilution, fragmentation and production of acid metabolites with a lower weight than normal, which compromises the homeostasis. [33] Therefore, for improvement of TMJ symptoms and function, it is necessary to remove the catabolites from the inflammation by lavage and to maintain the effect with exogenous SH and physiotherapy exercises. This could be more effectively done if the pain was suitably controlled in the early periods, as occurred in our study, with significant pain improvement by day 28 in the viscoelastic supplemented group.

In conclusion, an i.a. injection of SH following arthroscopic lysis and lavage is effective in reducing the pain in patients with TMJ dysfunction, this being statistically significant by day 14 after surgery, and so it could be used to aid normal post-surgical physiotherapy. Furthermore, treatment with SH maintains its analgesic effect in the long term (6 months), justifying post-arthroscopic use. Also, unlike in other previous studies, it has been demonstrated that the results of SH viscoelastic supplementation enhance arthroscopy, as arthroscopic lysis and lavage is already a technique with a great therapeutic effect in treating TMJ dysfunction.

These results encouraged us to continue with the prospective follow-up of the patients of our hospital in the following years. Thus we have been able to obtain information from a larger number of patients than in the pilot study.

After the finished study, arthroscopic procedures have been formalized by means of the use of SH in a systematic protocol in our hospital in all the surgical procedures, independently of the Wilkes stage, for all the patients who were coming to our service and were diagnosed of TMJ dysfunction without response to conservative measures. For this reason, in the last year we have treated by arthroscopy with SH infiltration 22 additional patients with TMJ disorder, who were including Wilkes stages III, IV and V. A follow-up of 6 months was carried out in all patients.

New obtained results have shown a statistically significant reduction (p<0.01) in joint pain compared to baseline. TMJ pain decreased from a mean value of 51,82mm above 100 in the analogical visual scale at baseline to 31,59mm in the last visit. Regarding the analysis of the maximum mouth opening variable, the initial mean value was 32,68mm, increasing significantly to 38,55mm in the last visit. The improvements were maintained over the 6-month follow-up period.

These results together with a very good tolerance of the product and no adverse effects during the follow-up of the patients, confirm us the evidence of the information obtained in the previous pilot study (J Oral Maxillofac Surg 68:1069-1074, 2010).

Recent findings suggest similar conclusions for the use of SH in TMJ disorders [34,35] and some studies showed that viscosupplementation with hyaluronic acid injections has an additional value with respect to joint lavage alone (arthroscopy, arthrocentesis). [36,37] This could verify if arthroscopy and SH have a positive effect on the signs of joint degeneration. [38]

All the data reaffirm us in the combined treatment of arthroscopic surgery plus SH in the TMJ dysfunction for its safety and optimum therapeutic effect.

REFERENCES

[1]   McCain JP, Sanders B, Koslin MG, et al: Temporomandibular joint arthroscopy: a 6-year multicenter retrospective study of 4.831 joints. *J. Oral Maxillofac. Surg.* 50:926, 1992.

[2]   Zingg M, Iizuka T, Geering AH, et al: Degenerative temporomandibular joint disease: surgical treatment and long-term results. *J. Oral Maxillofac. Surg.* 52:1149, 1994.

[3]   Kirk WS, Calabrese DK: Clinical evaluation of physical therapy in the management of internal derangement of the temporomandibular joint. *J. Oral Maxillofac. Surg.* 47:113, 1989.

[4]   Okeson JP: Long-term treatment of disk-interference disorders of the temporomandibular joint with anterior repositioning occlusal splints. *J. Prosthet. Dent.* 60:611, 1988.

[5]   Nitzan DW, Dolwick MF, Martinez GA: Temporomandibular joint arthrocentesis: a simplified treatment for severe, limited mouth opening. *J. Oral Maxillofac. Surg.* 49:1163, 1991.

[6]   Kurita K, Goss AN, Ogi N, et al: Correlation between preoperative mouth opening and surgical outcome after arthroscopic lysis and lavage in patients with disc displacement without reduction. *J. Oral Maxillofac. Surg.* 56:1394, 1998.

[7]   Smolka W, Iizuka T: Arthroscopic lysis and lavage in different stages of internal derangement of the temporomandibular joint: correlation of preoperative staging to arthroscopic findings and treatment outcome. *J. Oral Maxillofac. Surg.* 63:471, 2005.

[8]   Dimitroulis G: A review of 56 cases of chronic closed lock treated with temporomandibular joint arthroscopy. *J. Oral Maxillofac. Surg.* 60:519, 2002.

[9]   White RD: Arthroscopic lysis and lavage as the preferred treatment for internal derangement of the temporomandibular joint. *J. Oral Maxillofac. Surg.* 59:313, 2001.

[10]   Bertolami CN, Gay T, Clark GT, et al: Use of sodium hyaluronate in treating temporomandibular joint disorders: a randomized, doble-blind, placebo-controlled clinical trial. *J. Oral Maxillofac. Surg.* 51:232, 1993.

[11] Oliveras-Moreno JM, Hernandez-Pacheco E, Oliveras-Quintana T, et al: Efficacy and safety of sodium hyaluronate in the treatment of Wilkes stage II disease. *J. Oral Maxillofac. Surg.* 66:2243, 2008.

[12] Guarda L, Tito R, Staffieri A, et al: Treatment of patients with arthrosis of the temporomandibular joint by infiltration of sodium hyaluronate: a prelimirary study. *Eur. Arch. Otorhinolaryngol.* 259:279, 2002.

[13] Sato S, Ohta M,Ohki H, et al: Effect of lavage of sodium hyaluronate for patients with nonreducing disk displacement of temporomandibular joint. *Oral Surg. Oral Med. Oral Pathol. Oral Radiol. E*ndod. 84:241, 1997.

[14] Sato S, Goto S, Kasahara K, et al: Effect of pumping with injection of sodium hyaluronate and the other factors related to outcome in patients with non-reducing disk displacement of the temporomandibular joint. *Int. J. Oral Maxillofac. Surg.* 30:194, 2001.

[15] Alpaslan GH, Alpaslan C: Efficacy of temporomandibular joint arthrocentesis with and without injection of sodium hyaluronate in treatment of internal derangements. *J. Oral Maxillofac. Surg.* 59:613, 2001.

[16] Kopp S, Carlsson GE, Haraldson T, et al: Long-term effect of intra-articular injections of sodium hyaluronate and corticosteroid on temporomandibular joint arthritis. *J. Oral Maxillofac. Surg.* 45:929, 1987.

[17] Guarda-Nardini L, Masiero S, Marioni G: Conservative treatment of temporomandibular joint osteoarthrosis: intra-articular injection of sodium hyaluronate. *J. Oral Rehabil.* 32:729, 2005.

[18] McCain JP, Balazs EA, De la Rua H: Preliminary studies on the use of a viscoelastic solution in arthroscopic surgery of the temporomandibular joint. *J. Oral Maxillofac. Surg.* 47:1161, 1989.

[19] Mancha de la Plata M, Muñoz-Guerra M, Escorial-Hernandez V, et al: Unsuccessful temporomandibular joint arthroscopy: is a second arthroscopy an acceptable alternative? *J. Oral Maxillofac. Surg.* 66:2086, 2008.

[20] Sanders B, Buoncristiani R: Diagnostic and surgical arthroscopy of the temporomandibular joint: clinical experience with 137 procedures over a 2-year period. *J. Craniomandib. Disord.* 1:202, 1987.

[21] Holmlund AB, Axelsson S, Gynther GW: A comparison of discectomy and arthroscopic lysis and lavage for the treatment of chronic closed lock of the temporomandibular joint: a randomized outcome study. *J. Oral Maxillofac. Surg.* 59:972, 2001.

[22] Clark GT, Moody DG, Sanders B: Arthroscopic treatment of temporomandibular joint locking resulting from disc derangement: two-year results. *J. Oral Maxillofac. Surg.* 49:157, 1991.

[23] Indresano AT: Arthroscopic surgery of the temporomandibular joint: report of 64 patients with long-term follow-up. *J. Oral Maxillofac. Surg.* 47:439, 1989.

[24] Mosby EL: Effects of temporomandibular joint arthroscopy. A retrospective study. *J. Oral Maxillofac. Surg.* 51:17, 1993.

[25] Moses JJ, Sartoris D, Glass R, et al: The effects of arthroscopic lysis and lavage of the superior joint space on TMJ disc position and mobility. *J. Oral Maxillofac. Surg.* 47:674, 1989.

[26] Murakami KI, Tsuboi Y, Bessho K, et al: Outcome of arthroscopic surgery to the temporomandibular joint correlates with stage of internal derangement: five year follow-up study. *Br. J. Oral Maxillofac. Surg.* 36:30, 1998.

[27] Nitzan D, Dolwick MF, Heft MW: Arthroscopic lavage and lysis of temporomandibular joint: A change in perspective. *J. Oral Maxillofac. Surg.* 46:798, 1990.

[28] Dimitroulis G, Dolwick MF, Martinez A: Temporomandibular joint arthrocentesis and lavage for the treatment of closed lock: a follow-up study. *Br. J. Oral Maxillofac. Surg.* 33:23, 1995.

[29] Hirota W: Intra-articular injection of hyaluronic acid reduces total amounts of leukotriene C4, 6-keto-prostaglandin F1alpha, prostaglandin F2alpha and interleukin-1beta in synovial fluid of patients with internal derangement in disorders of the temporomandibular joint. *Br. J. Oral Maxillofac. Surg.* 36:35, 1998.

[30] Neo H, Ishimaru JI, Kurita K, et al: The effect of hyaluronic acid on experimental temporomandibular joint osteoarthrosis in the sheep. *J. Oral Maxillofac. Surg.* 55:1114, 1997.

[31] Balazs EA: Analgesic effect of elastoviscous hyaluronan solutions and the treatment of arthritic pain. *Cells Tissues Organs* 174:49, 2003.

[32] Miyazaki K, Gotoh S, Okawara, et al: Studies on analgesic and anti-inflammatory effects of sodium hyaluronate (SPH). *Pharmacometrics* 28:1123, 1984.

[33] Yeung R, Chow R, Samman N, et al: Short-term therapeutic outcome of intra-articular high molecular weight hyaluronic acid injection for nonreducing disc displacement of the temporomandibular joint. *Oral Surg. Oral Med. Oral Pathol Oral Radiol. Endod.* 102:453, 2006.

[34] Manfredini D, Bonnini S, Arboretti R, Guarda-Nardini L: Temporomandibular joint osteoarthritis: an open label trial of 76 patients treated with arthrocentesis plus hyaluronic acid injections. *Int. J. Oral Maxillofac. Surg.* 38:827-834, 2009.

[35] Long X, Chen G, Cheng AH, et al: A randomized controlled trial of superior and inferior temporomandibular joint space injection with hyaluronic acid in treatment of anterior disc displacement without reduction. *J. Oral Maxillofac. Surg.* 67:357-361, 2009.

[36] Manfredini D, Piccotti F, Guarda-Nardini L: Hyaluronic acid in the treatment of TMJ disorders: a systematic review of the literature. *Cranio* 28(3):166-76, 2010.

[37] Guarda-Nardini L, Ferronato G, Favero L, et al: Predictive factors of hyaluronic acid injections short-term effectiveness for TMJ degenerative joint disease. *J. Oral Rehabil.* 38(5):315-20, 2011

[38] El-Hakim IE, Elyamani AO: Preliminary evaluation of histological changes found in a mechanical arthropatic temporomandibular joint (TMJ) exposed to an intra-articular Hyaluronic acid (HA) injection, in a rat model. *J. Craniomaxillofac. Surg. Epub.*, Jan, 2011.

In: Arthroscopy   ISBN: 978-1-61470-955-8
Editors: K. Elani et al.   © 2012 Nova Science Publishers, Inc.

Chapter VI

Office-Based Knee Arthroscopy Using a Scope for Small Joints

Ken Okazaki, Hiromasa Miura, [*]
Shuichi Matsuda, and Yukihide Iwamoto
Department of Orthopaedic Surgery,
Graduate School of Medical Sciences,
Kyushu University, Maidashi, Higashi-ku, Fukuoka, Japan

ABSTRACT

Although arthroscopy has a low degree of invasiveness, it still requires considerable time, cost, and effort to be perfomed in the operating room. Surgeons or patients sometimes hesitate due to risks and constrains, especially for a diagnostic second-look arthroscopy. In order to make knee arthroscopy less invasive, we use a 1.9 mm–diameter scope. The purpose of this study is to assess the feasibility and usefulness of this method for diagnostic knee arthroscopy without using the operating room. Local anesthesia is placed at the lateral infrapatellar portal, and the joint is inflated. Skin and capsule are penetrated directly by the apex of the obturator, and the scope is inserted into the joint. Saline irrigation is used during arthroscopic evaluation. The wound is closed by a bandage,

[*] Address correspondence to: Hiromasa Muira, MD, PhD. Department of Orthopaedic Surgery, Graduate School of Medical Sciences, Kyushu University, 3-1-1, Maidashi, Higashi-ku, Fukuoka, 812-8582 Japan. Tel: 092-642-5860. Fax: 092-642-5507.E-mail: miura@med.kyushu-u.ac.jp.

without need for suture. Video images obtained during arthroscopy were reviewed by three orthopaedic surgeons. The images were scored based on the classification from three categories: 3 points, useful; 2 points, somewhat useful; 1 point, useless. The average point was used for the final evaluation. The patients assessed pain with a visual analog scale (100 mm long from no pain [0] to unbearable pain [100]). Twenty patients were reviewed on this cliteria. Video images were evaluated as 3 points for fifteen patients, as 2.7 points for three and 2.3 points for two patients. Mean pain score was 13.4 mm. Downsizing the scope allows the procedure to be done simply as insertion and removal without incision or suture, reducing risk of infection. This technique makes diagnostic arthroscopy feasible in the office of clinic without using the operating room and increases the likelihood of direct observation of the joint whenever the surgeon or patient feels it necessary. Thus, this method is especially useful for second-look diagnosis of cartilage in settings such as post-cartilage repair.

Keywords: arthroscopy, out-patient clinic, office-based surgery, follow-up, minimally invasive

HISTORICAL PERSPECTIVE

Arthroscopic evaluation remains a reliable method for assessment of joint disorders despite remarkable progress in imaging technology including magnetic resonance imaging (MRI). Arthroscopy provides better information in evaluation of surface cartilage than MRI [1]. However, arthroscopy is invasive and time-consuming; it is usually performed in the operating room, consuming time and staff effort [2]. In some cases where arthroscopic evaluation would probably be the best diagnostic method, surgeons and patients sometimes hesitate to accept the operating room constraints and risks of an invasive operative procedure. For instance, although second-look arthroscopy is useful to evaluate treatment results for cartilage injury, arthroscopy may only be done in practice if residual symptoms exist.

To overcome logistical and risk-related constraints on use of diagnostic arthroscopy, we assessed the feasibility of using a thin arthroscope for diagnostic evaluation of the knee. Because the small-joint arthroscope (diameter, 1.9 mm) is as thin as a 18-gauge needle, the procedure does not require any incision or suture, which makes the arthroscopic evaluation less invasive and less associated with risks such as infection [3, 4]. Downsizing of arthroscope makes the procedure feasible on the couch in the office of outpatient clinic without using the operating room. The purpose of this study is to ascertain whether the arthroscope of 1.9 mm diameter provides a useful view and to assess the feasibility of arthroscopy in the clinic office.

INDICATIONS AND CONTRAINDICATIONS

Because the area that can be observed is smaller than that obtained with conventional arthroscopy, usage of the new technique should be limited to cases in which the location of the lesions is known. Therefore, diagnosis of a cartilage lesion is the best indication for this method. For example, the second-look observation of cartilage injuries previously treated by mosaicplasty, fixation of cartilage fragment, or microfracture technique is a good indication. In these cases, MRI had not provided satisfactory information. Based on the clear view from arthroscopy, the surgeon could make informed decisions on whether to allow each patient to return to sports activities or work. The follow-up for the autologous chondrocyte implantation would also be a good indication of this method because repetitive arthroscopy is possible, if needed. It is, however, difficult to probe joint structure with this method. We consider that if the surgeon plans to make another portal for instruments, the surgery should be performed in the operating room to reduce the risk of infection [3].

PREOPERATIVE PLANNING

The surgeon should know the location of lesions. If the lesion is located on the medial compartment, the arthroscope should be inserted at the medial portal.

TECHNIQUE

The patient is placed on the couch in a supine position in the office of the outpatient clinic. The knee is draped with aseptic technique, and local anesthesia is introduced at the infrapatellar portal with 1% lidocaine containing epinephrine. The joint is also inflated with 30 ml of 0.5% lidocaine. The arthroscope used is 1.9 mm in diameter and 4.0 cm long (Karl Storz

Endoskopy Gmbh and Co., Tuttlingen, Germany). The skin and capsule are directly penetrated by the apex of the obturator and the scope is inserted into the joint. The joint is irrigated with saline during arthroscopic evaluation. After evaluating the lesion, saline solution is dumped from the cannula and the wound is closed by a bandage.

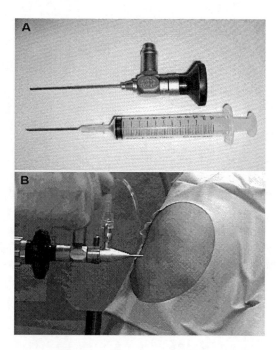

Figure 1. A. Small-joint arthroscope (diameter, 1.9 mm) and a syringe with 18-gauge needle. B. Use of 1.9 mm–diameter arthroscope. The skin and knee capsule were directly penetrated by the obturator with a cannula under local anesthesia, followed by scope insertion.

RESULTS

We assessed the usefulness of the obtained view and the affliction during the procedure in twenty patients (average age ± SD: 40.4 ± 16.9 years old). Eleven patients underwent second- or third-look arthroscopy for treatment of cartilage lesions. Four patients underwent diagnostic arthroscopy for cartilage injury, and five patients underwent second-look arthroscopy for reconstruction of anterior cruciate ligament. Table 1 shows patient characteristics.

Table 1. Patient characteristics

No	age	sex	Diagnosis and purpose	VAS	Image Evaluation
1	25	M	2nd look of previous mosaicplasty for osteochondritis dissecans	9	2.7
2	15	M	2nd look of previous fixation of osteochondritis dissecans	11	3
3	30	F	2nd look of previous microfracture for osteonecrosis	8	3
4	42	F	Diagnosis of cartilage injury	15	3
5	52	F	2nd look of previous microfracture for cartilage injury	22	3
6	22	M	2nd look of ACL reconstruction	10	2.3
7	48	M	Diagnosis of cartilage injury	14	3
8	53	F	3rd look of previous microfracture for cartilage injury	12	3
9	69	F	2nd look of previous microfracture for osteonecrosis	9	3
10	48	M	Diagnosis of cartilage injury	9	3
11	28	F	2nd look of ACL reconstruction	15	3
12	32	M	2nd look of ACL reconstruction	20	2.7
13	25	M	2nd look of ACL reconstruction	18	3
14	32	F	Diagnosis of cartilage injury	22	3
15	35	F	2nd look of previous microfracture for	9	3
16	20	M	cartilage injury	10	2.3
17	19	M	2nd look of previous mosaicplasty for	16	3
18	31	F	osteochondritis dissecans 2nd look of	11	3
19	36	F	previous fixation of osteochondritis dissecans	18	3
20	37	M	3rd look of previous microfracture for osteonecrosis 2nd look of previous mosaicplasty for cartilage injury 2nd look of ACL reconstruction	10	2.7

VAS, visual analog pain scale (0-100 mm); ACL, anterior cruciate ligament.
Image evaluation was the average point of gradings from 3 to 1 point (3, useful; 2, somewhat useful; 1, not useful) by three blinded, orthopaedic surgeons.

Four days after arthroscopy the patient was checked for any sign of infection. Pain during the procedure was assessed by a visual analog scale (VAS) (full length, 100 mm; 0=no pain, 100=unbearable pain). Video images obtained during arthroscopy were reviewed by three orthopaedic surgeons who were not engaged in this study. The images were scored based on the classification from three categories: 3 points, useful image; 2 points, somewhat useful image; 1 point, useless image. The average point was used for the final evaluation. The protocol of this study was reviewed and approved by the institutional review board and performed with the informed consent of the patients.

Duration of arthroscopic evaluation was usually only a few minutes. Video images were evaluated as 3 for fifteen patients, as 2.7 for three patients and as 2.3 for two patients. Mean pain score was 13.4 on the 100-mm scale (standard deviation: 4.6 mm, range: 8-22 mm). There were no complications, including local inflammation or wound infection.

CASE PRESENTATION

A 15-year-old boy had osteochondritis dissecans at his lateral femoral condyle. Arthroscopy was carried out with conventional method using a 4.5 mm-diameter arthroscope at the operating room.

The cartilage fragment was reduced and fixed with three bio-absorbable pins and three autologous osteochondral plugs subsequent to the arthrotomy (Figure 2A). His symptoms disappeared in 3 months, showing a full range of motion. Second-look arthroscopy was carried out using the 1.9 mm-diameter arthroscope at the treatment room of outpatient clinic seven months after the initial surgery (Figure 2B). The arthroscopic view provided excellent information about the cartilage surface. The patient allowed returning to the sports activities after the arthroscopic evaluation.

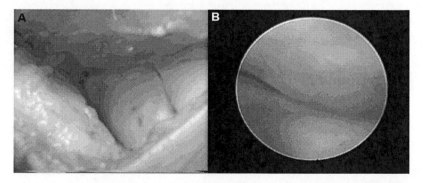

Figure 2. A. A 15-year-old boy had osteochondritis dissecans at his lateral femoral condyle. The cartilage fragment was reduced and fixed with three bio-absorbable pins and three autologous osteochondral plugs. B. Second-look arthroscopy was performed using the 1.9 mm–diameter scope seven months after surgery.

POSTOPERATIVE MANAGEMENT

The patient is allowed to return to normal activity soon after arthroscopy except for soaking in the bath for two days.

POSSIBLE CONCERNS, FUTURE
OF THE TECHNIQUE

Conventional arthroscopy is less invasive than open surgery and is often performed as a day procedure[5]. Even so, the conventional procedure using 4- to 5-mm scope requires small incisions and is usually performed in an operating room. Downsizing the diameter of the arthroscope to 1.9 mm eliminates the need for incisions and makes it possible to perform the procedure with a single extended action: insert, look and remove, which reduces the risk of infection. This minimally invasive procedure in our experience usually takes less than five minutes from puncture to the end. The wound is small and similar to those made by needle punctures performed daily in the outpatient clinic. Therefore, we conclude this procedure is feasible in the office of an outpatient clinic without using the operating room in the same way that the puncture of knee joint is done in the office. Performing arthroscopy on the couch in the clinic office reduces time and cost, and increases the likelihood of direct observation of the joint whenever the surgeon or patient feels it necessary.

We have an experience to use the other 1.9 mm–diameter arthroscope that has a fiber optic system. However, a better view can be obtained using an arthroscope with a lens system. Furthermore, the camera head should have a magnification lens.

In summary, we used a 1.9 mm–diameter arthroscope to evaluate the knee joints of twenty cases. This new technique is quick, easy and minimally invasive. It reduces risk of infection and makes diagnostic arthroscopy feasible in the outpatient clinic treatment room. The new method increases the chance of obtaining the best possible diagnosis based on direct vision at the bedside of the clinic office with no need to schedule the operation.

REFERENCES

[1]   Friemert B, Oberlander Y, Schwarz W, et al. Diagnosis of chondral lesions of the knee joint: Can mri replace arthroscopy? A prospective study. *Knee Surg. Sports Traumatol. Arthrosc.* 2004; 12: 58-64.

[2]   Forssblad M, Jacobson E, Weidenhielm L. Knee arthroscopy with different anesthesia methods: A comparison of efficacy and cost. *Knee Surg. Sports Traumatol. Arthrosc.* 2004; 12: 344-9.

[3]   Babcock HM, Carroll C, Matava M, et al. Surgical site infections after arthroscopy: Outbreak investigation and case control study. *Arthroscopy* 2003; 19: 172-81.

[4]   Jacobson E, Forssblad M, Weidenhielm L, et al. Knee arthroscopy with the use of local anesthesia--an increased risk for repeat arthroscopy? A prospective, randomized study with a six-month follow-up. *Am. J. Sports Med.* 2002; 30: 61-5.

[5]   Yoshiya S, Kurosaka M, Hirohata K, et al. Knee arthroscopy using local anesthetic. *Arthroscopy* 1988; 4: 86-9.

In: Arthroscopy   ISBN: 978-1-61470-955-8
Editors: K. Elani et al.   © 2012 Nova Science Publishers, Inc.

Chapter VII

Augmentation Technique with Hamstring Tendons in Chronic Partial Lesions of the ACL: Clinical and Arthrometric Analysis

R. Buda, *F. Di Caprio, R. Ghermandi,*
A. Ruffilli, ** *and A. Ferruzzi*
II Clinic of Orthopaedic and Traumatology, Istituto Ortopedico Rizzoli,
University of Bologna, Bologna, Italy

ABSTRACT

ACL (anterior cruciate ligament) partial tears include various types of lesions, and an high rate of these lesions evolve into complete tears. Most of the techniques described in literature for the surgical treatment of chronic partial ACL tears, don't spare the intact portion of the ligament. Aim of this study was to perform a prospective analysis of the results

* Corresponding Author: Phone: +39 051 6366212 Fax: +39 051 6366179 E-mail: roberto.buda@ior.it.
** Corresponding Author: Phone: +39 3471084968 Fax: +39 051 6366179 E-mail: aruffilli@tiscali.it.

obtained by augmentation surgery using gracilis and semitendinosus tendons to treat partial sub-acute lesions of the ACL. This technique requires an "over the top" femoral passage, which enables salvage and strengthening of the intact bundle of ACL. The study included 89 patients treated consecutively at our Institute from 1993 to 2003 with a mean injury-surgery interval of 21 weeks (12 - 39). Patients were followed up by clinical and instrumental assessment criteria at 3 months, 1 year and 5 years after surgery. Clinical assessment was performed with the IKDC form. Subjective and functional parameters were assessed by the Tegner activity scale. Instrumental evaluation was done using the KT-2000 instrument: the 30 pound passive test and the manual maximum displacement test were performed. We obtained good to excellent results in 96.6% of cases. We didn't observed recurrences in ligamentous laxity. We believe that the described technique has the advantage of being little invasive, compatible with the ACL anatomy, and enables very rapid functional recovery and return to sport.

INTRODUCTION

Partial lesions of anterior cruciate ligament (ACL), in particular in young active patients with very high functional demands, can evolve into complete tears [37] with significant knee instability. Reviewing the literature the rate of partial tears ranges from 28% [28] to 35% [24] of distortional traumas of the knee with hemarthrosis, and from 10 to 28% of all other ACL lesions [21]. 38% of partial lesions evolve into complete tears according to Noyes [29], whereas Fruensgaard et al. put this rate at 50% [13]. Danylchuk et al. [9] stated that partial ACL tears can evolve into complete because of interruption of blood vessels and thus necrosis of the intact fibers. The two most important elements that the orthopaedic surgeon should consider in order to chose the most adequate treatment (conservative or surgical) are the amount of initial ligament damage and the functional demand of the patient [29,31,42,43]. Conservative treatment relies principally on two methods: a rehabilitative protocol specific for muscular strengthening and proprioceptive recovery and the use of arthroscopic thermal shrinkage with radiofrequency [20,40,41]. In patients with low functional demand or in case of minor lesions of the ACL the first method can be effective. Thermal shrinkage is usefull to tighten up the ligament providing short time benefit, but high rate of failures are reported at long term follow-up [1,2,10,12,14,17,30,34,38,39].

In young active patients with a high functional demand, even after a conservative program, surgical treatment is often required, because of the persistence of symptomatic instability [3, 29]. When ACL reconstruction is required, a standard procedure is generally used, thus sacrificing the residual portion of the ACL. Reviewing the literature we didn't find any technique which considered the possibility to spare the intact portion of the ACL. In the last 15 years we have been using a surgical technique of augmentation with semitendinosus and gracilis tendon in the treatment of partial ACL tears [7]. This technique enables the intact portion of the ACL to be spared and provides a tendinous support structure that strengthens the residual portion of the ligament allowing an accelerated rehabilitation and a rapid return to sports. Aim of this contribution is to describe the surgical technique and to report the results obtained in a series of patients at 5 years follow-up.

MATERIALS AND METHODS

Eighty-nine patients with chronic unilateral partial ACL tear were consecutively treated between 1993 and 2003. Partial ACL tears were defined according to the clinical and arthroscopic criteria described by Barrack et al. [4]:

- Lachman test scores zero or 1+ (less than 5 mm);
- Pivot shift test is negative or only trace-positive;
- With diagnostic arthroscopy a significant portion of at least one bundle is healthy and is potentially functional as judged by palpation with a probe and arthroscopic anterior drawer testing.

In 23 cases the lesion involved the antero-medial band of the ACL, whereas in the remaining 66 cases it involved the postero-lateral band. With regards to associated lesions, in three cases there was a lesion of the posterior horn of the medial meniscus, in six cases a lesion of the posterior horn of the lateral meniscus, and in eleven cases a grade I–II chondropathy of the patello-femoral joint. All patients had no radiographic signs of knee joint degeneration, and they had healthy controlateral knees. Sixty of the 89 patients were men and 29 were women. Mean age was 24.7 years (range: 16–29). The mean injury–surgery interval was 21 weeks (range: 12–41). Before trauma, 47 patients were involved in competitive sports (soccer, basketball, volleyball, tennis, skiing), whereas the remaining 42 practiced recreational sports. Both groups were involved in high demanding sports activities. According to the

Tegner activity scale, the mean pre-injury sports activity level was 6.9 (range: 4–8). Before surgery, all patients underwent a non-standardized rehabilitation program for 8–12 weeks; after the rehabilitation program the patients were not able to resume their sports activity.

SURGICAL TECHNIQUE

Under general or peripheral anesthesia the patient was placed supine and a tourniquet was positioned.

Preliminary arthroscopic evaluation was performed by two standard portals (antero-lateral and antero-medial). The entire ACL was examined to assess the extent of ligament damage, with special attention to its proximal portion. Palpation of the residual ligament enabled mechanical strength to be assessed, while the anterior drawer maneuver performed under arthroscopic control provided a functional evaluation. During the arthroscopic examination, any combined intra-articular lesion was evaluated and eventually treated. In our series we performed chondral debridement of the patello-femoral joint in eleven cases, lateral release in three cases and partial meniscectomy in nine cases.

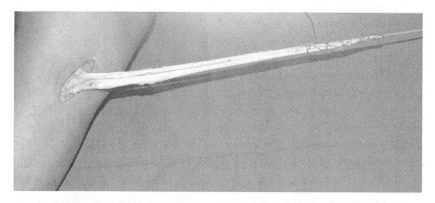

Figure 1. Preparation of the tendon graft. Semitendinosus and Gracilis tendons are harvested preserving the tibial insertion; the proximal third of the tendons is tacked with non reabsorbable suture.

Accurate cleaning of the periligamentous structures allowed the graft passage points to be identified and freed, both at the tibial and femoral level. A vertical incision in the proximal medial metaphysis of the tibia was made to isolate the semitendinosus and gracilis tendons. The tendons were harvested carefully with a tendon stripper preserving the tibial insertion. The proximal third of the two tendons was tacked with four non-reabsorbable suture threads (Ethibond n° 2), after removing the residual muscle tissue (Figure 1). The tibial tunnel was performed with a guide wire starting 5 mm medially and 5 mm superiorly to the bone insertion of the gracilis tendon. The emergence of the tibial guide wire in the joint was found close to the peripheral fibers of the residual portion of the ACL but is different for AMB (antero-medial bundle) and PLB (postero-lateral bundle). If the AMB had to be restored, the tibial tunnel was in the anatomic footprint of this bundle; in case of PLB reconstruction, the tibial tunnel emergence was just postero-lateral to the insertion of the AMB. The tibial tunnel was drilled using a 7 or 8 mm cannulated reamer, depending on the size of the graft. Then the intra-articular passage for the graft was identified between ACL and PCL at the level of the intercondylar notch: this passage was not dependent from the bundle which had to be reconstructed (Figure 2). Through this passage, the lateral surface of the distal femur was reached, where the tendon graft was anchored by two metal staples in an "over the top" position (Figure 3).

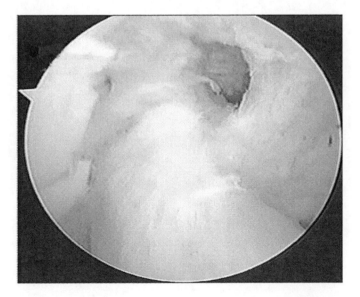

Figure 2. Arthroscopic view of the intra-articular passage of the tendon graft. The passage is not dependent from the bundle which had to be reconstructed and is identified between ACL and PCL at the level of the intercondylar notch.

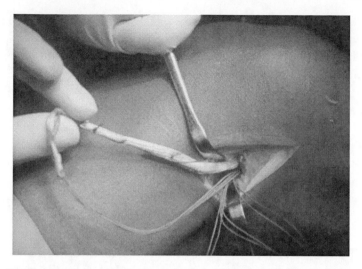

Figure 3. Fixation of the tendon graft on the lateral surface of the distal femur in an "over the top position".

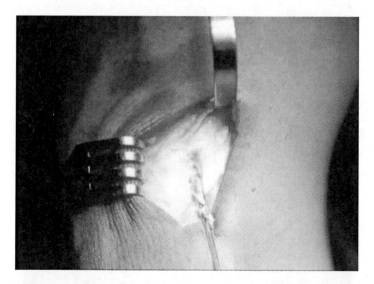

Figure 4. Fixation of the tendon graft, which was taken backwards anchored to a thread, by tenodesis on the anatomical insertion of the hamstring tendons.

The remaining portion of the tendons was taken backwards anchored to a thread and fixed by tenodesis on the anatomical insertion of the hamstring tendons (Figure 4). In case of AMB replacement, reconstruction is completely anatomic, with the graft placed in an 11 o'clock position, running parallel to the residual PLB (Figure 5). In case of PLB replacement, in order to save the residual AMB, the graft is not placed in a 10 o'clock; we had not an anatomic placement but we obtained a more vertical graft bridging and tensioning the AMB (Figure 6).

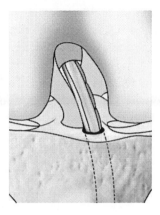

Figure 5. Reconstruction of the AMB. The intact portion of the ACL is preserved. The intra-articular emergence of the tibial tunnel is in the antero-medial region of the ACL insertion. The quadrupled hamstring graft is placed in the " over the top" position leaving intact its distal insertion. The graft is passed between the intact portion of the ACL and the PCL, in an 11 o'clock position.

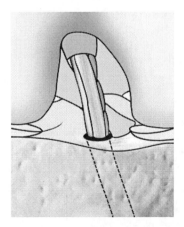

Figure 6. Reconstruction of the PLB. The intact portion of the ACL is preserved. The intra-articular emergence of the tibial tunnel is just postero-lateral to the insertion of the AMB. The quadrupled hamstring graft is placed in the " over the top" position leaving intact its distal insertion. The graft is passed between the intact portion of the ACL and the PCL.

POSTOPERATIVE TREATMENT

After surgery a rigid extension brace is worn overnight to avoid joint flexion contracture. The drainage is removed the day after surgery so that the patients is able to begin continuous passive motion (CPM): the degree of joint movement allowed on the first day is between 0° and 40° and can be increased according to the conditions and tolerance of the patient. Three days after surgery the patient is discharged and allowed to load the limb progressively, using the brace and two forearm crutches. The patient starts a home rehabilitation for the following 15 days. After 2 weeks full weight bearing is allowed without the brace. With the help of a physical therapist, the patient begins rehabilitation by performing closed chain kinetic exercises for the third and the fourth week; then open chain kinetic exercises are performed. Return to competitive sports is allowed 3 months after surgery.

PATIENT ASSESSMENT

Clinical assessment was performed by the IKDC score 3 months, 1 year and 5 years after surgery. The subjective and functional parameters were measured by the Tegner activity scale 1 and 5 years after surgery. Arthrometric instrumental assessment was carried out by KT-2000.

Table 1. IKDC and Tegner evaluation

IKDC	Repaired Bundle	Pre-op	3 months post-op	1 year post-op	5 years post-op
A	AMB	0	14	14	14
	PLB	0	43	48	47
B	AMB	15	8	8	8
	PLB	40	18	17	18
C	AMB	8	1	1	1
	PLB	26	4	1	1
D	AMB	0	0	0	0
	PLB	0	1	0	0
Tegner Activity Scale	AMB	6.7		6.3	6.1
	PLB	7.0		6.5	6.2

Table 2. KT 2000 post-operative and follow-up evaluation

Displacement (mm)	Post-operative	1 year	5 years
30 pounds displacement test (side to side difference)			
0-3	83	81	81
3-5	6	8	8
> 5	0	0	0
Manual maximum displacement test (side to side difference)			
0-3	78	77	77
3-5	11	12	12
> 5	0	0	0

The 30-pound passive test and manual maximum displacement test were performed postoperatively and 1 and 5 years after surgery. All data recorded at follow-up were analyzed statistically with the chi-square test and the Student's t test for independent data. P=0.05 was assumed as the significance cut-off.

RESULTS

At the final follow-up no case of re-rupture was observed. In seven patients surgery had to be repeated: in two cases to remove the staples in the lateral femoral condyle (2 and 3 years after surgery respectively); in two cases for a patellar lateral release (9 and 12 months after surgery respectively), and in three cases to perform a partial medial meniscectomy (2, 3 and 5 years after surgery respectively). Table 1 shows the results of the pre- and postoperative tests with the IKDC score and Tegner activity scale. We did not notice any difference in the overall results between the AMB and PLB reconstruction groups. The two cases classified as C by the IKDC score had knee pain, due to patello-femoral chondropathy in one case; in the other case a femorotibial chondropathy of the lateral compartment occurred, which produced joint effusions under stress which, however, did not prevent from amateur sports participation. In one case with an IKDC score of B, the patient complained of posterior pain in the tendon graft harvest site, due to retracting muscle scar. All patients regained full joint movement in extension, whereas there was a reduction in flexion of less than 5° in five patients. According to the Tegner Activity Scale the mean pre-lesional sports activity level was 6.9, whereas it was 6.5 1 year after surgery and 6.2 at the final follow up. None of the patients gave up with sports. Nine patients took up different sports for fear of re-injury. Eight patients resumed their previous sport at a lower level. The remaining 72 patients resumed their sport at previous level. There is not a statistically significant relationship between the age of patients and the time needed for return to contact sports participation. Table 2 shows the side-to-side difference in anterior tibial displacement with KT-2000. We had no complications, such as DVT or postoperative infection. In twelve patients in the immediate post-operative period we observed hematoma in the distal thigh, due to the tendon harvest, which resolved with rest and medical treatment.

DISCUSSION

Actually, the most common surgical technique performed to treat ACL lesions is the reconstruction using the semitendinosus and gracilis tendons.

Numerous authors proposed surgical techniques to attempt reconstructing the two-bundle anatomy of the ACL [7, 16, 18, 19, 25, 27, 33, 40, 44]. All these techniques require a single or even a double femoral tunnel. In the specific treatment of ACL partial tears, performing a femoral tunnel would mean to sacrifice the femoral origin of the intact portion of the ACL: an "over the top" femoral placement is the only possible technique if we want to spare this residual bundle. On the femoral side, in order to preserve the presence of the intact bundle of the ACL, the passage between the residual portion of the ACL and the PCL is the only one which can be used. If we have to reproduce a torn AMB, this passage allows us to place the graft in the 11 o'clock position (for the right knee), restoring the normal two-bundle anatomy of the ACL; but if we have to reconstruct the PLB, an anatomic passage of the graft is not permitted because of the presence of the intact AMB: in this case we have not an anatomic placement. Even on the tibial side, an anatomic placement is always possible for the reconstruction of the AMB; in PLB reconstruction the articular emergence of the tibial tunnel was not on the anatomic footprint of this bundle, but just lateral and posterior to the insertion of the intact AMB. This provides a more vertical graft placement, with the graft passing just in front of the AMB, with tensioning of the native AMB. The PLB is proven to have an important role when the knee is subjected to combined rotatory loads as produced for example in a pivot shift, and especially with the knee near full extension [15, 22, 26, 42, 45]: so an anatomic reconstruction of the PLB would be advised. A classical ACL reconstruction technique, which focuses primarily on reproducing the antero-medial bundle is proven to restore the antero-posterior stability [6, 15, 42]; moreover, classical single-bundle reconstruction techniques provided good long-term clinical results [5, 11, 32, 35, 36]. Secondly, in a partial ACL tear the rotatory instability is minimal or absent (the Pivot shift test is always negative or only trace positive), so we think that an anatomic reconstruction of the PLB is not strictly required in this case.

The most interesting aspect of this technique is that we have the possibility to spare the residual portion of the ACL and in our opinion this is important for various reasons:

(a) this assures mechanical strength in the immediate post-operative period, while the graft strength depends primarily on the fixation device: this allows an accelerated rehabilitation and a rapid return to sports;
(b) the residual portion maintains its blood supply, providing a support for the healing process in the graft [23];
(c) some proprioceptive innervation is maintained with evident benefits for the subjective outcome and for a safer return to sports.

In conclusion we think that the described technique is compatible with the ACL anatomy and provides good results thanks to the maintenance of the intact bundle, with its mechanical support and vessel and nerve supply representing an ideal solution for the treatment of chronic partial ACL tears in young and active patients.

REFERENCES

[1]   Andersson, C; Odensten, M; Good, L; Gillquist, J. Surgical or non surgical treatment of acute rupture of the anterior cruciate ligament: a randomized study with longterm follow-up. *J. Bone Joint Surg. Am.,* 1989, 71, 965–974.

[2]   Andersson, C; Odensten, M; Gillquist, J. Knee function after surgical or non surgical treatment of acute rupture of the anterior cruciate ligament: a randomized study with a long-term follow-up period. *Clin. Orthop.* 1991, 264, 255–263.

[3]   Bak, K; Scavenius, M; Hansen, S. et al. Isolated partial rupture of the anterior cruciate ligament. Long-term followup of 56 cases. *Knee Surg. Sports Traumatol. Arthrosc.,* 1997, 5, 66–71.

[4]   Barrack, RL; Buckley, SL; Bruckner, JD. et al. Partial versus complete acute anterior cruciate ligament tears. The results of nonoperative treatment. *J. Bone Joint Surg. Br.*, 72(4), 1990, 622–624.

[5]   Brandsson, S; Faxen, E; Kartus, J. et al. A prospective four- to seven-year follow-up after arthroscopic anterior cruciate ligament reconstruction. Scand. *J. Med. Sci. Sports,* 2001, 11, 23–27.

[6]   Brandsson, S; Karlsson, J; Sward, L. et al. Kinematics and laxity of the knee joint after anterior cruciate ligament reconstruction: pre- and post-operative radiostereometric studies. *Am. J. Sports Med.,* 2002, 30, 361–367.

[7]   Buda, R; Ferruzzi, A; Vannini, F; Zambelli, L; Di Caprio, F. Augmentation tecnique with semotendinous and gracilis tendon in chronic partial lesions of ACL: clinical and arthrometic analysis. *Knee Surg. Sport Traumatol. Artroscoc.,* 2006, Nov, 14 (11), 1101-7.

[8]   Caborn, DNM; Chang, HC. Single femoral socie double-bundle anterior cruciate ligament reconstruction using tibialis anterior tendon: description of a new technique. *Arthroscopy,* 2005, 21, 1273.e1–e8.

[9]   Danylchuk, KD; Finlay, JB; Krcek, JP. Microstructural organization of human and bovine cruciate ligaments. *Clin. Orthop.*, 1978, 131, 294–298.

[10]   Engebresten, L; Benum, P; Fasting, O. et al. A prospective, randomized study of three surgical techniques for treatment of acute ruptures of the anterior cruciate ligament. *Am. J. Sports Med.*, 1990, 18, 585–590.

[11]   Eriksson, K; Anderberg, P; Hamberg, P. et al. A comparison of quadrupled semitendinosus and patellar tendon grafts in reconstruction of the anterior cruciate ligament. *J. Bone Joint Surg. Br.*, 83, 2001, 348–354.

[12]   Feagin, JA; Jr, Curl, WW. Isolated tear of the anterior cruciate ligament: 5-year follow-up study. *Am. J. Sports Med.*, 1976, 4, 95–100.

[13]   Fruensgaard, S; Johannsen, HV. Incomplete ruptures of the anterior cruciate ligament. *J. Bone Joint Surg. Br.* 71(3), 1989, 526–530.

[14]   Freuensgaard, S; Kroner, K; Riis, J. Suture of the torn anterior cruciate ligament: 5-year follow-up of 60 cases using an instrumental stability test. *Acta Orthop. Scand.*, 1992, 63, 323–325.

[15]   Gabriel, MT; Wong, EK; Woo, SLY. et al. Distribution of in situ forces in the anterior cruciate ligament in response to rotatory loads. *J. Orthop. Res.,* 2004, 22, 85–89.

[16] Girgis, FG; Marhall, JL; Monajem, ARSA. The cruciate ligaments of the knee joint. Anatomical, functional and experimental analysis. *Clin. Orthop.,* 1975, 106, 216–231.

[17] Halbrecht, J. Long-term failure of thermal shinkage for laxity of the anterior cruciate ligament. *Am. J. Sports Med.,* 33(7), 2005, 990–995.

[18] Hamada, M; Shino, K; Horibe, S. et al. Single- versus bisocket anterior cruciate ligament reconstruction using autogenous multiple stranded hamstring tendons with EndoButton femoral fixation: a prospective study. *Arthroscopy,* 2001, 17, 801–807.

[19] Hara, K; Kubo, T; Suginoshita, T. et al. Reconstruction of the anterior cruciate ligament using a double bundle. *Arthroscopy,* 2000, 16, 860–864.

[20] Indelli, PF; Dillingham, MF; Fanton, GS. et al. Monopolar thermal treatment of symptomatic anterior cruciate ligament instability. *Clin. Orthop.,* 2003, 407, 139–147.

[21] Jacquot, L; Selmi, TAS; Servien, E. et al. Le'sions ligamentaires re'centes du genou. In: Encyclope'die medicochirurgicale appareil locomoteur. *Editions Scientifiques et Me'dicales Elsevier SAS Paris,* 2003, 14–080-A-20.

[22] Kanamori, A; Woo, SLY; Ma, CB. et al. The forces in the anterior cruciate ligament and knee kinematics during a simulated pivot shift test: a human cadaveric study using robotic technology. *Arthroscopy,* 2000, 16, 633–639.

[23] Krueger-Franke, M; Siebert, CH; Schupp, A. Refixation of femoral anterior cruciate ligament tears combined with a semitendinosus tendon augmentation. Technique and results. *Arch. Orthop. Trauma Surg.,* 1998, 117(1–2), 68–72.

[24] Liljedahl, SO; Lindvall, N; Wetterfors, J. Early diagnosis and treatment of acute ruptures of the anterior cruciate ligament; a clinical and arthrographic study of forty-eight cases. *J. Bone Joint Surg. Am.,* 1965, 47(8), 1503–1513.

[25] Marcacci, M; Molgora, AP; Zaffagnini, S. Anatomic double-bundle anterior cruciate ligament reconstruction with hamstrings. *Arthroscopy,* 2003, 19, 540–546.

[26] Markolf, KL; Burchfield, DM; Shapiro, MM. et al. Combined knee loading states that generate high anterior cruciate ligament forces. *J. Orthop. Res.,* 1995, 13, 930–935.

[27]   Muneta, T; Sekiya, I; Yagishita, K. et al. Two-bundle reconstruction of the anterior cruciate ligament using semiendinosus tendon with EndoButtons: operative technique and preliminary results. *Arthroscopy*, 1999, 15, 618–624.

[28]   Noyes, FR; Bassett, RW; Grood, ES. et al. Arthroscopy in acute traumatic hemarthrosis of the knee. Incidence of anterior cruciate tears and other injuries. *J. Bone Joint Surg. Am.*, 1980, 62(5), 687–695, 757.

[29]   Noyes, FR; Mooar, LA; Moorman, CT. III et al. Partial tears of the anterior cruciate ligament. Progression to complete ligament deficiency. *J. Bone Joint Surg. Br.*, 1989, 71(5), 825–833.

[30]   Odensten, M; Lysholm, J; Gillquist, J. Suture of fresh ruptures of the anterior cruciate ligament: a 5-year follow-up. *Acta Orthop. Scand.*, 1984, 55, 270–272.

[31]   Odensten, M; Hamberg, P; Nordin, M. et al. Surgical or conservative treatment of acutely torn anterior cruciate ligament: a randomized study with short-term follow-up observations. *Clin. Orthop.*, 1985, 198, 87–93.

[32]   Patel, JV; Church, JS; Hall, AJ. Central third bonepatellar tendon-bone anterior cruciate ligament reconstruction: a 5 year follow-up. *Arthroscopy*, 2000, 16, 67–70.

[33]   Pederzini, L; Adriani, E; Botticella, C. et al. Double tibial tunnel using quadriceps tendon in anterior cruciate ligament reconstruction. *Arthroscopy*, 2000, 16, E9.

[34]   Perry, JJ; Higgins, LD. Anterior and posterior cruciate ligament rupture after thermal treatment. *Arthroscopy*, 2000, 16, 732–736.

[35]   Pinczewski, LA; Deehan, DJ; Salmon, LJ. et al. A fiveyear comparison of patellar tendon versus four strand hamstring tendon autograft for arthroscopic reconstruction of the anterior cruciate ligament. *Am. J. Sports Med.*, 2002, 30, 523–536.

[36]   Ruiz, AL; Kelly, M; Nutton, RW. Arthroscopic ACL reconstruction: a 5–9 year follow-up. *Knee*, 2002, 9, 197–200.

[37]   Sandberg, R; Balkfors, B. Partial rupture of the anterior cruciate ligament. Natural course. *Clin. Orthop.*, 1987, 220, 176–178.

[38]   Sekiya, JK; Golladay, GJ; Wojtys, EM. Autodigestion of a hamstring anterior cruciate ligament autograft following thermal shrinkage: a case report and sentinel of concern. *J. Bone Joint Surg.*, 2000, 82-A, 1454–1457.

[39] Sherman, MF; Lieber, L; Bonamo, JR. et al. The longterm follow-up of primary anterior cruciate ligament repair. Defining a rationale for augmentation. *Am. J. Sports Med.*, 1991, 19, 243–255.

[40] Takeuchi, R; Saito, T; Mituhashi, S. et al. Double-bundle anterior cruciate ligament reconstruction using bone-hamstring-one composite graft. *Arthroscopy*, 2002, 18, 550–555.

[41] Thabit, G. III The arthroscopic monopolar radiofrequency treatment of chronic anterior cruciate ligament instability. *Op. Tech. Sports Med.*, 1998, 6, 157–160.

[42] Woo, SL-Y; Kanamori, A; Zeminski, J. et al. The effectiveness of reconstruction of the anterior cruciate ligament with hamstrings and patellar tendon. A cadaveric study comparing anterior tibial and rotational loads. *J. Bone Joint Surg. Am.*, 2002, 84, 907–914.

[43] Yao, L; Gentili, A; Petrus, L. et al. Partial ACL rupture: an MR diagnosis?. *Skeletal. Radiol.*, 1995, 24(4), 247–251.

[44] Yasuda, K; Kondo, E; Ichiyama, H. et al. Anatomical reconstruction of the antero-medial and postero-lateral bundles of the anterior cruciate ligament using hamstring tendon grafts. *Arthroscopy*, 20, 1015–1025.

[45] Yasuda, K; Kondo, E; Ichiyama, H. et al. Surgical and biomechanical concepts of anatomic anterior cruciate ligament reconstruction. *Oper. Tech. Orthop.*, 2005, 15, 96–102.

In: Arthroscopy
Editors: K. Elani et al.

ISBN: 978-1-61470-955-8
© 2012 Nova Science Publishers, Inc.

Index

E

F

T